OXFORD MEDICAL PUBLICATIONS

Hospital Referrals

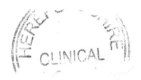

OXFORD GENERAL PRACTICE SERIES

Editorial Board

3. Preventive medicine in general practice
   edited by J.A.M. Gray and G.H. Fowler
5. Locomotor disability in general practice
   edited by M.I.V. Jayson and R. Million
6. The consultation: an approach to learning and teaching
   D. Pendleton, P. Tate, P. Havelock, and T. Schofield
8. Management in general practice
   P.M.M. Pritchard, K.B. Low, and M. Whalen
9. Modern obstetrics in general practice
   edited by G.N. Marsh
10. Terminal care at home
    edited by R. Spilling
11. Rheumatology for general practitioners
    H.L.F. Currey and S. Hull
12. Women's problems in general practice
    (Second edition)
    edited by Ann McPherson
13. Paediatric problems in general practice
    (Second edition)
    M. Modell and R.H. Boyd
14. Epidemiology in general practice
    edited by D. Morrell
15. Psychological problems in general practice
    A.C. Markus, C. Murray Parkes, P. Tomson, and M. Johnston
16. Research methods for general practitioners
    David Armstrong, Michael Calnan, and John Grace
17. Family problems
    Peter R. Williams
18. Health care for Asians
    B.R. McAvoy
19. Continuing care: the management of chronic disease
    (Second edition)
    edited by J.C. Hasler and T.P.C. Schofield
20. Geriatric problems in general practice
    (Second edition)
    G.K. Wilcock, J.A.M. Gray, and J.M. Longmore
21. Efficient care in general practice
    G.N. Marsh

Hospital Referrals

Oxford General Practice Series • 22

Edited by

MARTIN ROLAND and ANGELA COULTER

OXFORD   NEW YORK   TOKYO
OXFORD UNIVERSITY PRESS
1992

Oxford University Press, Walton Street, Oxford OX2 6DP

Oxford New York Toronto
Delhi Bombay Calcutta Madras Karachi
Petaling Jaya Singaprore Hong Kong Tokyo
Nairobi Dar es Salaam Cape Town
Melbourne Auckland

and associated companies in
Berlin Ibadan

Oxford is a trade mark of Oxford University Press

Published in the United States
by Oxford University Press, New York

A catalogue record for this book is available from the British Library

Library of Congress Cataloging in Publication Data
Hospital referrals / edited by Martin Roland and Angela Coulter.
(Oxford general practice series; 22) (Oxford medical publications)
1. Medical referrals. 2. Medical referrals — Great Britain.
3. Hospitals — Utilization. 4. Hospitals — Great Britain
— Utilization. I. Roland, M. O. (Martin Oliver) II. Coulter,
Angela. III. Series. IV. Series: Oxford general practice series; no. 22.
[DNLM: 1. Family Practice — methods. 2. Referral and Consultation. W1 OX55 no. 22]
R727.5.H67   1992   362. 1 — dc20   92–19067
ISBN 0–19–262174–2 (paperback)

Typeset by
Graphicraft Typesetters Ltd, Hong Kong
Printed in Great Britain by Bookcraft (Bath) Ltd
Midsomer Norton, Avon

Preface

There are number of reasons why general practitioners' referrals to hospital have become a subject of great interest in recent years. The general practitioner has acted as gatekeeper to the hospital service since the inception of the National Health Service, as the great majority of patients attending hospitals are referred there by their general practitioner. Over the last decade, a number of studies have emphasized the wide variation in referral patterns that exists among general practitioners, with some sending four or five times as many patients to hospital as their colleagues. The reasons for this variation remain unclear. Against this background, the recent changes to the management structure of the NHS have meant that all aspects of health care have come under scrutiny to see whether the most effective use is being made of available resources. Since GPs seem to vary so greatly in the frequency with which they refer, it is not surprising that hospital referrals have become of considerable interest to politicians and purchasers of health care.

In editing this book, we have attempted to cover the majority of areas which we believe to be important in relation to hospital referral at the present time, and we have tried to address the varying perspectives of different groups who have an interest in hospital referral. The majority of chapters in the book have practical orientation. We hope that general practitioners will be interested in the chapters on how to collect and analyse referral data, how to audit referrals, how to improve communication with consultants and how to develop referral guidelines. The book will also be of interest to hospital consultants, particularly those chapters describing ways of improving communication with general practitioners, whether by developing better standards of written communication or by meeting to discuss referral guidelines. We hope that the two chapters on developing and evaluating referral guidelines will encourage general practitioners and consultants to consider meeting to discuss local referral policies, which we believe is a particularly valuable way to take forward discussion about how to derive greatest benefit from referrals. We have not attempted to cover purely clinical areas or to define which medical problems should be referred to hospital.

The book should also be of interest to public health physicians and to health service managers, particularly those with responsibility for purchasing health care. These groups need to understand how data on hospital referrals can be collected, how to interpret variability, and how to assess the effectiveness of the referral process. While GPs, specialists and managers all have their own perspective on referrals, it is the patient for whom care is being planned or provided, and it was therefore essential also to include a chapter on the patient's perspective. We also sought to set the book in a broader context by including a chapter on the historical development of the referral system, and a chapter on how primary care physicians refer to specialists in other countries of the world.

Most of the authors have carried out recent research in the areas about which they are writing, and most of the chapters are extensively referenced. The book arrives at a time when general practitioners will have received some feedback from their Family Health Services Authorities on the referral data contained in their first Annual Reports, and we hope that the book will contribute constructively to the debate about how hospital facilities may be used most effectively.

March   M.R.
1992   A.C.

Contents

Contributors

David Armstrong   Reader in Medical Sociology, United Medical and Dental Schools of Guy's and St. Thomas's Hospitals

Angela Coulter   Deputy Director, Health Services Research Unit, Department of Public Health and Primary Care, University of Oxford

Douglas Fleming   Director, Birmingham Research Unit of the Royal College of General Practitioners

Jeremy Grimshaw   Wellcome Research Fellow, Department of General Practice, University of Aberdeen

Andrew Haines   Professor of Primary Health Care, University College and Middlesex School of Medicine

Roger Jones   Professor of Primary Health Care, The Medical School, University of Newcastle upon Tyne

Nigel Oswald   Director of Studies in General Practice, School of Clinical Medicine, University of Cambridge.

Martin Roland   Professor of General Practice, The Medical School, University of Manchester

Ian Russell   Director, Health Services Research Unit, University of Aberdeen

Barry Tennison   Director of Information, Cambridge Health Authority

David Wilkin   Associate Director, Centre for Primary Care Research, Department of General Practice, University of Manchester

1 The interface between primary and secondary care

Angela Coulter

Introduction — Why are referrals important?

Referral to a specialist clinic is one of the options open to a general practitioner when deciding how best to help a patient. The referral may be only one of many actions taken during the course of an episode of illness. On average, a British GP with 2000 patients on his or her list can be expected to make about 240 referrals per year (RCGP/OPCS/DHSS 1986). This may seem a trivial amount in the context of a GP's total annual workload of around 7000 consultations. Why then are referrals important?

This book has been compiled in the belief that referrals are both important and informative. They are important because the decision to refer is rarely straightforward; the referral can be problematic at the individual clinical level, but it also has economic, social, and political implications because the referral system is the gateway to hospital care. The decisions made in general practice are crucial determinants of the use of health service resources. An understanding of referral patterns is vital for planning hospital and other health service facilities. Furthermore, the strength of general practice in the British medical hierarchy can be said to depend, at least in part, on the existence of the referral system.

Referrals are informative because of what they reveal about the way in which the health service works. By examining the history and development of the referral system we can learn about relationships between the various professional groups involved in health care delivery and how these relationships have changed over time. By comparing the British referral system with those in other countries we can learn much about the factors governing health policy in various parts of the world. Detailed examination of the outcomes of referral decisions can provide the basis for achieving improvements in the quality of care. Above all, study of the referral system raises crucial questions about medical decision-making and the scientific basis of medical knowledge.

Until the reorganization of the UK National Health Service (NHS) in 1991 there were no routine data systems collecting information about GPs' referrals or use of outpatient facilities. However, in the early 1970s information began to emerge from a series of research studies which suggested that there were wide variations in the rates at which GPs referred patients to specialist clinics. Later studies using more sophisticated techniques of data collection and analysis confirmed the early impression that rates were variable, but failed to identify any factors which could explain the major sources of variation. Meanwhile, a separate strand of research examined rates of admission to hospital and found that these also exhibited considerable variation, both between countries and between small areas within countries (McPherson *et al.* 1982). For the most part the research reflected the organizational split between primary and secondary care, in which outpatient referrals and inpatient admissions were considered in isolation from each other. More recently, researchers have begun to explore relationships between referrals and admissions (Coulter *et al.* 1990).

The realization that there were large unexplained variations in the likelihood of being referred to a specialist or admitted to hospital was disturbing from a number of points of view. Although this was further evidence of geographical inequalities in access to and use of health services, the variations in referral and admission rates could not be explained by geographical differences in resource levels and they did not appear to be related to differences in morbidity rates or to levels of patient demand. This pointed to differences in the way clinical decisions are made as being the key determinants of the variations. The notion that doctors' views on how best to treat patients could vary to such an extent seriously undermined the popular view of medicine as a coherent, scientifically-based activity (Andersen and Mooney 1990). In order to appreciate how it is that such different patterns of practice can arise, we need to examine the structure of the referral system and the mechanisms underlying the decision to seek specialist involvement in patient care.

Although the basic referral system is fairly straightforward, understanding the way in which it works in practice is more complex. The research on which our knowledge of the referral system is based has involved the use of a variety of methodologies drawn from the toolbox of health services research. These range from qualitative studies of how decisions are made, through practical audits conducted in individual practices, to statistical analysis of data sets involving large numbers of GPs and their patients. Interpretation of the patterns observed has drawn on psychological, sociological, and economic theory to explain what is going on. The result of all this research has been an increased awareness of the variations inherent in clinical practice and a new focus on the need for evaluation in order to establish good practice guidelines.

How does the referral system work?

A referral system can be defined as the organizational structure for referring medical problems from generalists to specialists. Typically this involves patients referred by their GPs to the outpatient clinics of hospital consultants. In urgent cases GPs can refer patients for inpatient admission to hospital, although this occurs much less frequently than outpatient referral. GPs can also refer to a variety of other practitioners, including physiotherapists, speech and occupational therapists, clinical psychologists, chiropodists, dieticians, community psychiatric nurses, social workers, and so on. Usually a GP making a referral will write a letter to the consultant or department concerned giving details of the patient and their current problem, and the patient will then be asked to attend the relevant clinic at an appointed time. Following the initial outpatient consultation the patient may be discharged back to the care of their GP, they may be given further appointments in the outpatient clinic, or they may be placed on a waiting-list for admission to hospital.

GPs are not the only practitioners who can make referrals. Patients are often cross-referred from one consultant clinic to another, or they may be asked to attend the outpatient clinic following an inpatient admission. There are a number of other health care professionals who can sometimes initiate outpatient referrals. As examples, clinical medical officers can refer patients to paediatric, ENT, or eye clinics; health visitors can refer to hearing clinics, eye clinics, or to child psychiatry; orthoptists can refer to eye clinics; and social workers can refer to child psychiatry.

In Britain the referral system is fairly tightly controlled; with few exceptions, specialists will not see patients unless they have been initially referred by a doctor or one of the health professionals mentioned above. However, patients do have a right of self-referral to hospital accident and emergency departments. These departments are intended to cater for trauma and other emergencies, although some patients use casualty departments inappropriately for non-urgent primary care. There are certain other cases in which patients have a right of direct access to a specialist department; for example, genito–urinary clinics usually operate an open-door policy, as do clinics for drug and alcohol abuse.

Patients who have private health insurance, or those who opt to pay directly for consultations, also rely on referral from their GP to the private clinics of specialists. Private health care is on the increase in Britain. In 1966 less than 3 per cent of the UK population had some form of private health insurance cover (Central Statistical Office 1990). By the end of 1990 this proportion had risen to 13 per cent (7.6 million people) (Health Service Journal 1991).

Most of the population insured privately use a combination of NHS and private health care. Private general practice is relatively rare, and most patients rely on the NHS for trauma or emergency care. The greatest use of private health care by the insured population is in elective surgery. In 1986 17 per cent of patients undergoing elective surgery were treated in the private sector. The private surgery rate was very unevenly distributed throughout the country, ranging from 6 per cent of all elective surgery

performed in the Northern Regional Health Authority area to 31 per cent
in North West Thames (Nicholl *et al.* 1989).

Patients may ask to be referred privately in order to avoid long
waiting-times for outpatient consultation or inpatient admission. Admission to a private bed can secure better hotel facilities and greater privacy.
Private admissions may be to independent hospitals catering only for
private patients, or to private wards within NHS hospitals. Some patients
having been referred to NHS outpatient clinics may decide to switch to
private facilities if the specialist decides to admit them to hospital. The
opposite combination sometimes occurs as well, when the patient is
referred to a private outpatient clinic but eventually is admitted to an
NHS bed.

There are some situations when the referral system can be bypassed, in
addition to those mentioned above. Patients who have been seen in an
outpatient clinic may sometimes be able to go back there without seeing
their GP first. As examples, patients with skin problems may be given
freedom to phone the clinic for an appointment if their condition
deteriorates, and patients who have attended a rheumatology clinic may
make further appointments when their joints flare up. This type of access
is often time-limited. A consultant may tell a patient to make appointments directly for six months, but to contact his or her GP thereafter.
Even without a formal arrangement, patients who have seen a consultant
may simply telephone if they experience further problems, and be given a
further appointment in this way. This occurs particularly when patients
with chronic diseases get to know a consultant quite well over a period of
years. However, these arrangements may be discouraged as health care
purchasing becomes more sophisticated, and fundholding GPs may be
reluctant to pay for outpatient consultations which have not been
sanctioned by them.

Who gets referred?

Not surprisingly perhaps, the likelihood of being referred to a specialist
outpatient clinic is strongly related to age. It is also related to sex. Figure
1.1 shows the rate of referral by age-group and sex from data recorded by
36 practices in the Oxford Region in 1990/1 (Bradlow *et al.* 1992).

The patterns were different for males and females. Women were more
likely to be referred than men in all but the youngest and oldest age
groups, with high rates of referral in the middle years. Referrals to
obstetric clinics were excluded from these data, so pregnancy does not
account for the high rate of referral among women between the ages of 25
and 54. However, we do know that women are more likely to consult their
GPs in these age-groups and the referral patterns mirror consultation
rates quite closely (OPCS 1991).

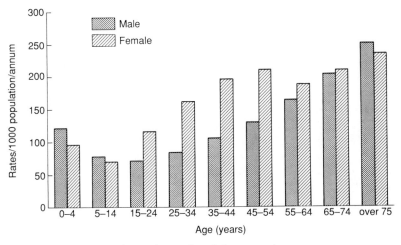

Fig. 1.1 Outpatient referrals by sex and age group.

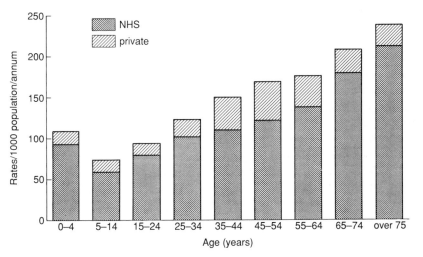

Fig. 1.2 Type of referral by age group.

Out of the total of 45 617 outpatient referrals in this 1990/1 study, 20 per cent went to private clinics, reflecting the relatively high rate of use of private health care among the population living in the Oxford Regional Health Authority area. There was considerable variation between practices in the proportion referred privately, ranging from 5–50 per cent. Middle-aged patients were more likely to be referred privately than those in the youngest and oldest age-groups (Fig. 1.2). This probably reflects patterns of employer-subsidized private health insurance, and the fact that elective surgery is more common in this age-group.

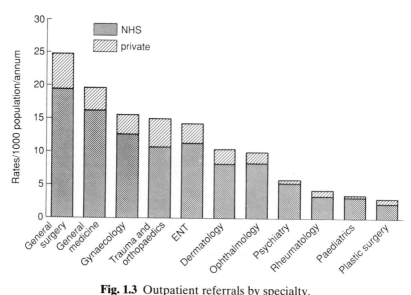

Fig. 1.3 Outpatient referrals by specialty.

The distribution of outpatient referrals by specialty is shown in Fig. 1.3. General surgery attracted the greatest number of referrals, followed by general medicine, gynaecology, trauma and orthopaedics, and ENT. Private referrals were most common to clinics in general surgery and orthopaedics, and least common for paediatrics and psychiatry.

Figure 1.4 shows the ten problems which figured most commonly among the outpatient referrals recorded in the Oxford study. Pain in the joints, abdomen, and back were common precipitating factors for the referrals recorded in this study. Two conditions experienced exclusively by women — breast lumps, and menorrhagia or heavy periods — featured in the top ten problems, contributing to the high rate of referral among middle-aged women. Requests for sterilization (vasectomy and female sterilization) were common, as were requests for treatment for varicose veins and for hearing aids. Skin disorders and vision disturbances also featured among the top ten problems, which accounted for 20 per cent of all outpatient referrals.

Where do GPs refer?

In theory British GPS have always been free to refer their patients to any hospital or consultant clinic in the country. In practice there have been some limitations to this freedom, increasingly so in recent years. The 1990 NHS and Community Care Act, which introduced the internal market in health care, required purchasers of health care to agree contracts with

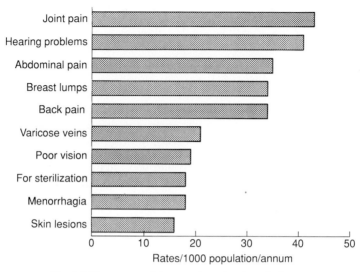

Fig. 1.4 Top ten problems referred to hospital.

providers. Practices which opted to become fundholders (when they were given a budget from which to purchase outpatient services and elective surgical procedures) were free to agree contracts with any units to which they wished to refer, but non-fundholders wanting to refer to hospitals with which their district health authority (DHA) did not have a contract had to seek the approval of district officials. At the time of writing these extracontractual referrals (ECRs) have attracted a considerable amount of media attention, but it is too early to assess the extent to which the traditional freedom of referral is being eroded. The government's stated aim was to develop a system which was responsive to GPs' preferences. The Department of Health (1989) stated that 'The object is to secure the referral patterns which local GPs wish to see put in place unless there are compelling reasons for not doing so.'

DHAs were told to consult with local GPs to identify their preferred referral patterns. This was no easy task since there were no routine data available on current patterns and there was no tradition of involving GPs in health service planning. Indeed, staff in regional health authorities (RHAs) and DHAs, who had had no direct responsibility for general practice prior to the 1990 Act, were often ignorant of the particular concerns of GPs, and the family health services authorities (FHSAs), which had recently taken on major new responsibilities, were still in the process of developing their management and planning capacity.

There are several factors which can influence a GP's choice of referral location. These include:

(1) geographical location — most referrals go to the general hospital nearest to the practice, but the nearest hospital may not be in the district where the patient is resident;

(2) transport — for some patients the availability of public transport may be more important for access than the proximity of the hospital;

(3) waiting-times — if GPs are provided with accurate information about waiting-times for outpatient appointments or inpatient admissions then this may influence their choice of hospital;

(4) preferred consultant — it is usual to refer to a named consultant (in the 1990/1 Oxford study cited above, 93 per cent of referrals went to a named consultant), so a GP's knowledge of consultants may govern the choice of hospital;

(5) technical facilities — the availability of particular facilities may be a relevant factor;

(6) patient preference — patients may have their own reasons for wanting to be referred to a particular hospital.

Practices vary widely in the range and number of referral locations used. A study conducted in 1983/4 of referrals from 32 practices in the Oxford RHA found that over a 12-month period, practices referred to an average of nine different hospitals or units (Coulter *et al.* 1989). While one practice sent all their referrals to only four locations, another referred to 42 different units. The majority of the referrals (79 per cent of a total of 17 691) went to NHS clinics in the district in which the practice was located, a further 9 per cent went to other districts within the same region, 2 per cent went to NHS clinics outside the Oxford RHA, and 10 per cent went to private hospitals and clinics. Patterns were similar in the second Oxford study conducted seven years later in 1990/1; the rate of private referral was higher, but the proportion referred outside the RHA boundaries remained very small (Bradlow *et al.* 1992).

Why do GPs refer?

There are a variety of reasons for referring patients to specialist outpatient clinics. These include referral for diagnosis or for an investigation which cannot be done by the GP, referral for advice on the best means of treating the patient's condition, referral for the specialist to initiate a course of treatment, and referral for a second opinion or to reassure the patient. These are the commonly accepted instrumental reasons for referring patients to specialist clinics. However, sometimes there are other more subtle reasons which may not be openly acknowledged, but which may nevertheless be important influences on the decision to refer. Factors which may precipitate referral include a GP's perceived need for a specialist to share the load of treating a difficult or demanding patient; a deterioration in the GP/patient relationship leading to a desire by either party to involve someone else in managing the problem; a concern to involve a specialist prompted by fear of malpractice litigation; or direct requests by patients or their relatives.

Sometimes these reasons are not communicated to the specialist to whom the referral is made, which can lead to misunderstanding of the GP's and patient's expectations. Studies have shown that the three parties to the referral — GP, specialist, and patient — sometimes have very different views about the appropriateness of referral decisions. One of the problems with the referral system as it operates at present is the failure to clarify the objectives of each individual referral, and this problem seems to be fairly common.

Some commentators have argued that GPs have unique referral thresholds (Cummins *et al.* 1981; Morrell *et al.* 1971). Since no one has succeeded in demonstrating a relationship between referral rates and easily measured factors which might have been expected to influence them (i.e. case-mix; patient characteristics such as age, sex, and social class; or practice characteristics such as list size, number of partners, or type of premises — see Chapter 6) it may be more fruitful to seek explanations for the variations in referral patterns by examining the psychology of medical decision-making. Factors inherent in the person-ality of individual GPs, such as their willingness to tolerate uncertainty or to take risks, their personal enthusiasms, and their perceptions of the availability and benefits of treatment, may combine to create a particular referral threshold (Wilkin and Dornan 1990). However, it is likely that external factors associated with health care organization and resourcing, together with social pressures from professional colleagues, patients and their relatives, as well as the particular practice styles of individual GPs, all exert an influence on referral decisions.

What information do we have about referral patterns?

GPs' referral patterns have been the subject of research for some considerable time. Early studies were concerned with documenting rates and patterns and as early as 1953 Logan noted 'startling differences' between the referral rates in eight practices (Logan 1953). Hopkins (1956) described the variety of reasons for referring patients to hospital, report-ing that 54 per cent were for treatment, 31 per cent were for diagnosis or investigation, and 15 per cent were for consultant opinion and advice. Fry (1959) reported that only 3.8 per cent of his patients had been referred to specialist outpatient clinics during the course of 1957, although 13 per cent had been referred for X-ray or pathology investigations. The four conditions he referred most commonly were acute disk lesions, haemor-rhoids, the 'acute abdomen', and hernias. Fry's patients were referred to specialist clinics primarily for treatment (73 per cent).

Since then the volume of published literature on referral rates and patterns of referral has grown considerably. It is now the most heavily researched aspect of the interface between primary and secondary care (Wilkin and Dornan 1990). On average GPs make about 5 referrals per 100 consultations, or about 12 referrals per 100 registered patients per year. All studies have found that rates vary between GPs and between practices. Estimates of the extent of variation between individual GPs themselves vary, partly because of the difficulty in establishing a correct denominator (Chapter 5), but it is fairly well established that rates vary between practices by at least threefold or fourfold (Wilkin and Smith 1987; Noone *et al.* 1989).

According to the General Household Survey the proportion of the population consulting a GP in the two weeks prior to the survey rose from 12 per cent in 1981 to 15 per cent in 1989 (OPCS 1991). However, the proportion of consultations resulting in a referral has remained the same throughout this period at around 13 per cent of patients consulting.

Data from the National Morbidity Study suggest that practices' referral rates are remarkably consistent. Eighteen practices participated in both the first study in 1970–1 and the third study in 1981/2. There was a strong positive correlation between the referral rates in these two surveys, despite the large inter-practice variability (Crombie and Fleming 1988).

Prompted by the 1991 NHS reorganization, which increased the need for health authorities (HAs) to monitor referral patterns, computerized systems are being installed in hospitals that will facilitate routine data collection and analysis. From 1st April 1991 all outpatient clinics were required to collect a minimum data set of information in a standardized form. This includes national GP and practice codes and the source (whether the patient was referred by a GP, by an accident and emergency department, by another hospital consultant, or self-referred). When this system is fully implemented it should be possible for the first time to identify referrals from individual practices to individual hospitals. In theory it should also be possible to aggregate information about referrals across a number of hospitals or units. Since some referrals cross DHA and RHA boundaries, it will be necessary to establish a national system of data exchange to track NHS referrals. Even then those referrals which go to independent hospitals — a substantial proportion in the case of some practices — will be missed unless private hospitals can be persuaded to participate in the data collection exercise.

In the meantime, the responsibility for collecting data on referrals rests with general practices, which are now required to include the information in their annual reports to FHSAs. There are numerous problems inherent in interpreting referral data collected in this way (Coulter *et al.* 1991), but it seems certain that referral rates and patterns will continue to be the focus of attention for some time to come. However, if the quality of referrals is to improve, it will be important to shift the focus from referral rates to assessments of the appropriateness of referrals.

How do you judge the quality of referrals?

Ideally each referral should meet the following criteria:

(1) it should be necessary for the particular patient, in the light of their presenting symptoms, age, previous treatment, and so on;

(2) it should be timely, i.e. neither too early nor too late in relation to the course of the disease;

(3) it should be effective, i.e. the objectives of the referral are achieved and the benefits outweigh the costs.

Since the patient may have a different view of the benefit to be gained from referral to that of the GP or the specialist, any assessment of appropriateness should take account of the patient's views as well as those of doctors. Ideally, patients should not be unduly inconvenienced as a result of referral so issues to do with the process of care, such as waiting-times, facilities in outpatient clinics, and the attitudes and behaviour of doctors and hospital staff, are also important quality indicators.

Other indicators of the quality of referrals include the communication of information from GPs to specialists, and vice versa, and the extent to which patients' views are elicited and taken into account when deciding on the most appropriate course of action. There is substantial evidence that GPs' referral letters and consultants' replies often fail to provide an adequate channel of communication (Wilkin and Dornan 1990; Chapter 8). Little is known about the extent to which patients are actively involved in decisions about their care, although we do know that they often have different priorities from those of doctors, and failure to determine these may result in sub-optimal outcomes (Chapter 9).

It is important in selecting patients for referral to ensure that all those who require specialist attention do indeed receive it. Referral rates are unsatisfactory indicators of appropriateness, because they can hide failures to refer as well as referrals made unnecessarily (Wilkin *et al.* 1989; Chapter 6). Patients may be harmed if referral occurs too late and delay leads to more major treatment being required at a later stage. Too great an emphasis on reducing referral rates may be counterproductive in the long run.

What are the advantages and disadvantages of the British system?

The system which pertains in Britain is by no means the only way of organizing access to health services. In many other countries patients have direct access to specialists (Chapter 3) as well as the ability to move freely between primary care practitioners, and foreign visitors are often surprised by the relative lack of freedom for patients here. The referral system amounts to a restrictive trade practice, brought in initially to protect the interests of doctors (Chapter 2), in which GPs have a monopoly on primary medical care and patients' autonomy is diminished. However, it does have a number of major advantages (Marinker 1988). Marinker lists the benefits relating to medical logic, to cost effectiveness, to the development of a rational hospital service, and to the place of general practice in UK society.

The first advantage is the role played by the GP as gatekeeper to expensive high-technology specialist care. The role ensures that the majority of care is contained within general practice, and that when specialist care is necessary the professional skill of the GP should ensure that this is directed to the most appropriate specialist at the most appropriate time. Furthermore, argues Marinker, the system of registering patients with one general practice results in the creation of a single comprehensive life-long record of the patient's health and care, which is indispensable for logical medical management.

The British referral system undoubtedly contributes to the relatively low cost of health care in this country. Marinker estimated that the cost of a consultation with a specialist in an outpatient clinic was four times that of a GP consultation. Since many of the problems seen in general practice fall within the province of several specialties, the absence of the generalist gatekeeper function could result in a huge increase in the number of cross-referrals from specialist to specialist. Also, since specialists depend to a much greater extent on expensive technology for investigation and treatment, costs could escalate dramatically if the use of specialist care increased. The referral system, according to Marinker, 'contributes to the improvement of the quality of care by limiting over-medicalization, over-investigation, and over-treatment'.

However, we need reassurance that the British system does not result in underinvestigation and undertreatment. Can we be sure that by containing the majority of care in the hands of generalists, British patients are not being deprived of specialist medical care from which they could benefit? Furthermore, the evidence that referral rates vary so much suggests that the benefits of specialist care are unevenly distributed. We need to be certain that patients' needs are being met as equitably as possible and that effective treatment is available as and when it is needed.

Marinker concludes that 'abolition of the referral system would be likely not only to damage general practice and the quality of health care; it would erode the functions of the NHS'. If we are to accept this argument, we must be sure that the system is working as well as it should.

Conclusion

The referral system is a key feature of the British health service. An understanding of the way in which it functions is essential for clinicians, managers, planners and health services researchers. In order to plan or evaluate a health system it is essential to understand the way in which patients gain access to the various health facilities. Studies of variations in referral patterns have demonstrated that clinical need is not the only factor determining access to specialists. Although the British system of referral from GPs to specialists has many advantages, there have been suggestions that it is not operating as efficiently as it might. The rest of this book aims to describe the current state of the referral system, as well as offering suggestions for improving it to ensure that it is worth defending.

References

Andersen, T.F. and Mooney, G. (1990) *The challenges of medical practice variations*. Macmillan Press, London.

Bradlow, J., Coulter, A., and Brooks, P. (1992). *Patterns of referral*. Health Services Research Unit, Oxford.

Central Statistical Office (1990). *Social Trends* **20**. HMSO, London.

Coulter, A., Seagroatt, V., and McPherson, K. (1990). Relation between general practices' outpatient referral rates and rates of elective admission to hospital. *British Medical Journal* **301**, 273–6.

Coulter, A., Noone, A., and Goldacre, M. (1989). General practitioners' referrals to specialist outpatient clinics: II. Locations of specialist outpatient clinics to which general practitioners refer patients. *British Medical Journal* **299**, 306–8.

Coulter, A., Roland, M., and Wilkin, D. (1991). *GP referrals to hospital: a guide for Family Health Services Authorities*. Centre for Primary Care Research, University of Manchester.

Crombie, D.L. and Fleming, D.M. (1988). General practitioner referrals to hospital: the financial implications of variability. *Health Trends* **20**, 53–6.

Cummins, R., Jarman, B., and White, P. (1981). Do general practitioners have different 'referral thresholds'? *British Medical Journal* **282**, 1037–9.

Department of Health (1989). *Contracts for health services: operational principles*. HMSO, London.

Fry, J. (1959). Why patients go to hospital: a study of usage. *British Medical Journal* **2**, 1322–7.

Health Service Journal (1991) Bumpy time for BUPA as the recession bites. *Health Service Journal* 11th July, 1991.

Hopkins, P. (1956). Referrals in general practice. *British Medical Journal* **2**, 873–7.

Logan, W.P.D. (1953). *General practitioners' records*. General Register office: Studies on medical and population subjects No. 7. HMSO, London.

Marinker, M. (1988). The referral system. *Journal of the Royal College of General Practitioners* **38**, 487–91.

McPherson, K., Wennberg, J., Hovind, O., and Clifford, P. (1982). Small-area variations in the use of common surgical procedures: an international comparison of New England, England and Norway. *New England Journal of Medicine* **307**, 1310–14.

Morrell, D., Gage, H., and Robinson, N. (1971). Referrals to hospital by general practitioners. *Journal of the Royal College of General Practitioners* **21**, 77–85.

Nicholl, J.P., Beeby, N.R., and Williams, B.T. (1989). Role of the private sector in elective surgery in England and Wales. *British Medical Journal* **298**, 243–7.

Noone, A., Goldacre, M., Coulter, A., and Seagroatt, V. (1989). Do referral rates vary widely between practices and does supply of services affect demand? *Journal of the Royal College of General Practitioners* **39**, 404–7.

Office of Population Censuses and Surveys (1991). *General Household Survey 1989*. HMSO, London.

Royal College of General Practitioners, Office of Population Censuses and Surveys, Department of Health and Social Security (1986). *1981–1982 Morbidity statistics from general practice: third national study*. HMSO, London.

Wilkin, D. and Dornan, C. (1990). *General practitioner referrals to hospital: a review of research and its implications for policy and practice*. Centre for Primary Care Research, University of Manchester.

Wilkin, D. and Smith, A. (1987). Variations in general practitioners' referral rates to consultants. *Journal of the Royal College of General Practitioners* **37**, 350–3.

Wilkin, D., Metcalfe, D.H., and Marinker, M. (1989). The meaning of information on GP referral rates to hospitals. *Community Medicine* **11**, 65–70.

2 The history and development of the referral system

Nigel Oswald

Introduction

For those of us who have only practised medicine under the NHS, a system of reference of problems from generalist to selected specialist seems natural, indeed obvious. However, in the past the process and activity of referral was surrounded by antagonism and anxiety, and in the 1990s referral seems set to become controversial again as, for the first time, doctors and civil servants offer their different interpretations of the apparently highly idiosyncratic referral behaviour of individual practitioners.

In order to understand the development of referral as we know it, it is essential to realize that up to 1947, when those establishing the NHS nationalized the hospitals and institutionalized the distinction between specialists and GPs, the business of referral was attended by anxieties and restrictions which we have forgotten, or of which we have never been aware. To understand this we need to go back to the tripartite origins of medical practice in the period before there was a medical 'profession' at all.

The medical profession

What we now regard as a unified profession began with three distinct types of practitioner, divided by education, social status, and income. These were the physicians, surgeons, and apothecaries. As we shall see later the equation of 'apothecary' and 'general practitioner' is simplistic. The three types of practitioner supplied different needs and fulfilled different functions, and did not regard each other as complementary parts of what could be termed a medical service.

The physicians, incorporated as a College by a Charter of Henry VIII in 1518, had a university education. The Fellowship of the College was confined to graduates of the Universities of Cambridge and Oxford, and therefore to members of the Anglican Church. Physicians were very largely of high, though not of the highest, social status. The Fellows claimed the right under their Charter to issue licences to others who wished to practise as physicians. The education of a physician was Classical and contained little that we would presently regard as medical. They diagnosed and gave a prognosis based on the patient's description of their illness and by observation of the appearance of the patient and their body fluids, chiefly urine. From these appearances it was thought possible to define the imbalance between the body's humours and propose how the balance be restored. Physical examination, with the exception of feeling the pulse, was not an activity undertaken by physicians, and did not form part of their diagnostic process until after the revolution in medical understanding which accompanied the French Revolution in the late eighteenth century. The physicians restricted their own numbers and were niggardly in the award of licences because their practice was with the well-to-do, of whom there was only a limited supply.

Tradesmen made a living by using their hands and the demeaning nature of physical contact with patients separated physicians from surgeons, whose origins extended back in time to man's first attempts to aid and heal fractures and wounds. Surgery was manual and, as such, at first unthinkable for those from the higher social classes. The treatment of ulcers and fractures, the incision of abscesses, and remedies for wounds of various kinds was the work of the surgeon. He was in demand at time of war, but otherwise he was generally unable to make an adequate living solely through other people's clumsiness and so required another trade, commonly as a barber, to make ends meet. The Association of Barber–Surgeons was founded in 1540, and this grew into the Royal College of Surgeons which was established in 1800, the connection with barbers having been abandoned on the way.

The physician, having diagnosed his patient, ordered a prescription. However, because of the stigma of trade, the rules of his College did not allow him to dispense it. This was the work of an apothecary. Apothecaries were in open competition for physicians' prescriptions and this led to some of the first conflicts over referral although the conflict was, to our eyes, reversed. Instead of free competition physicians and apothecaries sometimes made mutual agreements for a physician to use, and occasionally even employ, a particular apothecary. This was deeply resented by those not so favoured and was canvassed as an abuse through a number of cases in the sixteenth and seventeenth centuries. The reason for this is clear; although apothecaries existed to dispense the prescriptions of physicians, there were not enough physicians to provide a livelihood for more than a handful of apothecaries.

Apothecaries, being available to ordinary people in the streets of the towns, dispensed on their own account for those unable to afford the attention of a physician. Poor people and small tradesmen consulted apothecaries when unwell or in the case of sudden emergency and the number of apothecaries substantially exceeded that of physicians. During the plague of London in 1665 the physicians left London almost to a man.

The apothecaries stayed. This was not attributable to cowardice on the one hand or social conscience on the other. It merely reflected the fact that anyone rich enough left London, and their medical men went with them. The poor people stayed and therefore so did the apothecaries. The contrast between their behaviour was based on the different classes from whom they made their living.

The rules of the physicians' Charter gave them control over the apothecaries who were forbidden to compete with physicians by charging for medical advice, and were restricted to making a living by the sale of medicines, a fact which may still have reverberations in the expectations of patients and doctors to this day. The education of an apothecary was by apprenticeship. The ambiguity of their role as nominal dependents of the physicians and as physicians to the poor, coupled with their origins in the lower social classes, led to repeated conflicts over rights and status, especially with the physicians in London.

In the eighteenth century, therefore, the orthodox medical practitioners (I shall not consider the position of the healers and quacks) were apparently rigidly divided into three groups: university-educated physicians who diagnosed but did not dispense and confined their activities to patients from the higher social classes; apothecaries who dispensed for themselves and for physicians, confining their diagnostic skill to the lower classes and pretending, for legal purposes, that it did not exist; and the surgeons, carrying on a trade involving the supervision of any external manifestation of disease or injury, or any procedure involving cutting of the skin. Thus, in so far as the branches were truly separated, there was no place for referral as we know it. Patients referred themselves to the practitioner appropriate to their condition and social status. Referral between doctors is a phenomenon which became important only in the nineteenth century.

The historical evidence for the distinctions between the orthodox practitioners in their struggle for status is chiefly found in the records of their Colleges and Companies in London. There the concentration of population and the competition between the types of practitioner sharpened their distinctions and was emphasized particularly by the Royal College of Physicians which sought to dominate the others. Outside London the very small number of physicians and the difficulties of making a living ensured that in practice the distinctions between practitioners were much less clear cut than I have described. Kerrison (1814) stated that 'nineteen out of twenty' patients were treated by doctors who practised 'generally', i.e. within the territory of all three branches. Reduced to economic terms this meant that in order to make a living the practitioners, with the exception of a very small number in the largest centres of population, were obliged to take and treat any patients they could and, just as important, to retain them. Passing patients to other doctors was financial suicide, and this is the fundamental distinction separating the issues surrounding referral in the nineteenth and early twentieth centuries from the issues after the inception of the NHS.

In England only London was large enough to continuously support a population of doctors making a living as 'pure' physicians and 'pure' surgeons, and even in London that population was small. Elsewhere physicians dispensed, surgeons took on the role of physicians and also trespassed into the fields of the midwife and apothecary, and the apothecaries spread themselves in all directions. They did this because of a demand for their services and because their own economic survival demanded it. Doctors, and patients able to pay for medical care, were unevenly distributed, problems of transport and communication were almost unimaginable to us, and in the rural areas commonly none of the practitioners was available at all. Between 1750 and 1850 the group of surgeon–apothecaries gained greatly in strength (Loudon 1986) and licences from the College of Surgeons and the Society of Apothecaries (after the passing of the Apothecaries Act 1815) were frequently combined. The surgeon and apothecary, the 'physician in ordinary to most families', aspired to the trust and respect accorded to those with a university degree (Gregory 1772).

The medical acts

The first Medical Act was passed in 1858, setting up the General Medical Council and introducing a mechanism to distinguish qualified and unqualified practitioners. Definition of the standard of competence of practitioners was not attempted; all that was required was to pass an examination from one of the licensing bodies after completing an approved course of study.

The Medical Act of 1886 tackled the question of competence and specified for the first time that qualifying doctors must pass an examination in medicine, surgery, and midwifery, and that they must be proficient in the practice of all three branches at the time of qualification. Thus arose the concept that the purpose of medical education was the production of a competent GP. In the late nineteenth century this did not mean, as it came to mean in the 1950s, the GP competent to know when to refer, but the practitioner personally able to intervene effectively across the range of problems presented to him. Clinical diagnosis, surgical treatment, intervention in midwifery, and the dispensing of medicines were all, of necessity, within the range of ordinary practitioners, particularly in rural areas. It was assumed, and it was the reality, that referral to another practitioner would be a rare event.

However, a referral system did develop and is now fundamental to our practice of medicine. We must consider how this came about and how the conflicts between self-interest on the one hand and increasing specialism and technological advance on the other were resolved, and how, in the process, referral and its control became an important feature of medical ethics.

Paying patients

Right up until the advent of the NHS the fear of losing paying patients was a fundamental feature of the practice of all types of doctor. Many doctors, especially in their early years, struggled to survive financially. Patients who could and would pay for advice were few and far between, and the profits to be made from the sale of medicines were, in general, low. Many patients were simply unable to pay and it was pointless to expect them to do so. Many doctors took on heavy burdens of work under the Poor Law, because it was based on a modest but certain income, while they attempted to build up their practice of paying patients. Loudon (1986, p. 241) provides details of rates of pay and workload, which gradually deteriorated from the early to the middle nineteenth century. There were extreme examples, such as Mr Tatham of Huddersfield who, in 1843, received a salary of £40 as a Poor Law medical officer, out of which he bore the expense of the medicines supplied (an accepted arrangement). In his first year he made 1633 journeys and visits, dispensed medicines worth £37.18s.7d and made £2 on his year's work. Others were better paid, but Poor Law work was no way to make a fortune, or even a decent living.

Poor patients were expected to be grateful for any care they received, and they might not have access to a doctor at all. Paying patients might elect to consult another practitioner at any time. Their present doctor guarded them jealously and struggled to provide every service possible. Even when he was unable to do so referral was a rare event. Often there was no other practitioner more skilled than himself to consult and, where there was, frequently he also was struggling to thrive. There were many examples of physicians who, having been consulted for a second opinion, then adopted the role of GP for both patient and family (British Medical Journal 1878, 1906).

In 1886 this problem had become so widespread in London that it led directly to an attempt to establish an Association of General Practitioners who would agree to refer patients solely to consultants who stuck to consulting. A leader (British Medical Journal 1886*a*) stated that 'the consulting class do not hesitate to drop habitually into general practice and avail themselves of its material profits'. A circular letter to GPs in London was published in the same issue of the British Medical Journal and stated as an objective of the Association that 'the consultant should be applied to for advice by the practitioner, not the patient, and that the advice should be given for the instruction of the practitioner in the management of the case, and not for the instruction of the patient'

(British Medical Journal 1886*b*). The members pledged themselves 'to support, and support only, those distinguished members of the profession . . . who consult only with the profession and not with the public'.

The GPs, who were consulted by most of the population most of the time because of their availability and relatively modest fees, felt squeezed from all sides. They feared and risked losing patients to both specialists and hospitals, while at the same time medical developments ensured that both profession and patients recognized that treatment was becoming available which no practitioner could offer on his own.

The hospitals

We must remember that until the late nineteenth century hospitals were not generally regarded as houses of healing but as symbols of misery and destitution. Any procedure contemplated in the 1860s could be carried out as effectively in the patient's home as in hospital, provided he was well-off (Abel Smith 1964). Doctors and nurses were hired and a suitable room, temporarily converted, could at that time offer everything available in the operating theatres of a great hospital coupled with a substantially smaller risk of hospital-acquired infection. No one with means would go to a hospital under any circumstances. Entry to the voluntary hospitals of London and the provinces was on the basis of being a suitable object of charity, and commonly not for medical reasons. Entry to the workhouse infirmaries was on the basis of absolute destitution.

The voluntary hospitals were charitable institutions funded by endowments, subscriptions, and fundraising. A condition of entry was inability to afford care at home but the practice grew up that subscribers, for their contribution, expected the right to dispense 'their' charity and to admit needy dependents or petitioners to hospital for a period of care. This often had nothing to do with medical need, was not controlled by doctors, and was confined to people with certain kinds of conditions. Most hospitals would not admit children, infectious cases, or the chronic sick. If these people were so desperately needy as to be unable to be cared for by their own families they ended up in the workhouse infirmaries. These policies were not deliberately inhumane but represented a mixture of pragmatism (for example, in the exclusion of infectious people) coupled with an understanding of the purpose of a hospital very different from the current view.

However, advances in knowledge of the functioning of the body through the work of Bichat, Laennec, Dupuytren, Charcot, and many others in the aftermath of the French Revolution, coupled with, 50 years later, the introduction of anaesthesia and then the principles of antisepsis, meant that doctors came to regard hospitals as a resource for the study of illness, the education of students, and the practice of technical medicine.

This resulted in steadily increasing status for the better hospitals and for surgeons, in whose field the most spectacular advances were made.

From early times the Governors of voluntary hospitals had appointed a staff of medical men who gave their services to the charity. This in time became a stepping stone to building a private practice. To become known as physician or surgeon to a voluntary hospital was a sign of acceptance and an invitation to consultation. The staff, who excluded apothecaries, were also determined that appointments should be rigidly controlled and, especially in the London teaching hospitals, nepotism and snobbery were rife.

Attendance at the outpatient department of hospitals was by self-referral. Crowded and unpleasant as these were they were open to any person who attended and waited and there, as the status of the hospitals rose and the awareness of specialist expertise spread, patients who could afford to pay a practitioner would come in the knowledge that, if considered suitably interesting, a free specialist opinion and free admission and treatment could be obtained. The outpatient departments were controlled by 'house' staff, young doctors, usually protégés of members of the staff, who aspired one day to be appointed to the staff themselves. Gradually the idea grew up of using the outpatient department of great hospitals to supply interesting inpatient cases for treatment, teaching, and research. At the same time those aspirants who had developed skills in the departments, but could not gain appointments within the hospital or could not afford to continue to work for nothing, began to establish their own hospitals and advertise for patients with particular conditions — for example, of the eye or throat. These hospitals were not run as charities and catered for patients who would otherwise have been able to pay their practitioner, superseding the regular doctor by offering greater expertise.

In the absence of a formal referral system which prevented the 'poaching' of patients by specialists, and in the presence of a growing free service from provident dispensaries and from 'sick clubs' to which those who were poor but not destitute made weekly contributions, the GPs lived in a state of permanent anxiety.

Referral to consultants

The control of referral from practitioners to consultants and back was thus a highly contentious issue. Well into the twentieth century there was no clear-cut distinction between a group of doctors who functioned only as consultants and to whom it was safe to refer patients, and a group who were specialists but still prepared to care for more general and family problems, to whom it was not. The attempt to found an Association of GPs in 1886 had failed, but as a result of persisting difficulties in the first decade of the twentieth century the central ethical committee of the British Medical Association (BMA), which was now more effectively representing the views of GPs, produced a report (British Medical Journal 1908) which attempted to establish firstly, how a consultant should be defined, and secondly, what were the duties of consultant and practitioner after a referral had been made. The report was debated and accepted and went into considerable detail on such matters as who should precede whom into the sick room; the ordinary attendant was to enter before the consultant, and leave afterwards. The report boiled down to a statement that, if invoked as a consultant the specialist was placed in a position of trust in which ethical rules were broken if the consultant used the situation to obtain any lasting advantage or acted in a way which reduced the patient's confidence in their ordinary attendant.

As a sign of the fact that the hospital outpatient department had not, by 1908, become a significant venue for formal referral from practitioner to specialist, the report specifically stated that if consultation did not take place at the patient's home it would generally be at the home of the referring practitioner, who would arrange the time of the meeting. When the situation demanded, which meant a serious enough illness in a rich enough patient, prominent consultants would travel far and wide, a situation described by Trollope when the fictional Sir Omicron Pie travels by the Great Western Railway to offer a prognosis on the Dean of Barchester after his apoplexy. There can hardly be greater evidence of the change of medical life, comparing the consultant of 1900 travelling by carriage between his consulting rooms and the homes of well-off patients and today's consultants with their overcrowded hospital clinics and waiting-lists measured in months.

However, it is important to remember again that these concerns were largely those of the large towns and a small number of well-established consultants. More commonly, GPs worked to develop skills in a particular field and establish part of their practice on their reputation in it. In 1910 the BMA published another analysis of the relation between GPs and consultants, and identified doctors specializing in gout, radium, electricity, and X-rays, dietary therapy, and balneology (therapy by healing springs and waters) as intruding on the fields of GPs, physicians, and surgeons (British Medical Journal 1910). A specific complaint was that patients were choosing to consult practitioners who they believed to be more specialized and therefore superior in knowledge, but without the knowledge themselves to choose their specialist appropriately. Since GPs needed specialists and vice versa an uneasy accommodation, disturbed by temporary outbursts of resentment, was the pattern for referral during the late nineteenth and early twentieth centuries. The system which evolved was not governed by written rules but more by custom and etiquette.

National health insurance

The fact that this was a matter of balancing interests rather than of deep-rooted principle was proved by the introduction of Lloyd George's National Health Insurance Act of 1911 (NHI). In the 1880s the Prussians under Bismark had introduced an extensive, well-administered system of health insurance. In Britain it was gradually recognized that making it easier for working people to obtain medical care might benefit both them and the health of the nation, a point emphasized by the generally poor health of those called up for service in the Boer War.

A finely balanced scheme was introduced which covered working men, and would pay for the services of a GP but not for a specialist or for admission to hospital. The result was that practitioners, after widespread protests, came to think that it was in their interest to accept a 'panel' of patients for whom they would receive capitation fees whether they saw the patient or not, while continuing to derive traditional sources of income from better-off patients and from maternity work. Included in the provisions were some which militated against private referrals; for example, the fees of an anaesthetist would be deducted from the panel doctor's remuneration (Abel Smith 1964, p. 247). Thus the Act produced a considerable change in the attitude of practitioners to hospitals and their outpatient departments. The presence of a defined group of patients who had free access to a practitioner resulted in a substantial drop in out-patient attendances (Abel Smith 1964, p. 246, p. 333). At the same time capitation payments meant that the passing of more difficult cases to hospitals ceased to be so alarming.

The fact that specialist fees were not covered by NHI but a specialist opinion could be obtained free if patients were sent to outpatient depart-ments without detriment to practitioners' incomes encouraged GPs increas-ingly to refer patients to named hospital specialists and this, in time, resulted in a narrowing of GPs' skills, which was important in diminishing the status of general practice in the view of patients, specialists, and of practitioners themselves.

The First World War came later in the same decade. In this conflict many established practitioners joined the armed services. As a result practices were abandoned or left to locums, and the intense competition for patients between practitioners became particularly unsavoury as those who enlisted and risked their lives also saw their civilian livelihood wast-ing away.

The General Medical Council (GMC), which might have been in the forefront of the various controversies about the ethics and etiquette of referral, had allowed practice regarding the relationship between prac-titioners to depend on a gradual accumulation of 'generally recognised' behaviour. It is no coincidence that it was stung into making firm statements governing the subjects of advertising and canvassing for the first time in 1914. Strangely, there had been little previous interest from the body charged with overseeing doctors' professional conduct. Indeed, 35 years after its foundation, the Council was of the opinion (General Medical Council 1893) that there was no specific prohibition on advertising, although the activities of a small number of dental entrepreneurs made its members quite quickly change their minds. In 1905 the GMC had published warnings about what kind of action could be taken against practitioners who canvassed patients, especially if they deprecated the skills of another doctor, a warning which was aimed at both GPs and consultants. However, in a system without formal registration of patients it was difficult to draw a firm line between poaching patients and the patient's own right to a free choice of doctor, including specialists.

Thus in 1914 the GMC agreed and published a specific 'Warning Notice' which set out the situations in which a doctor might be guilty of serious professional misconduct (General Medical Council 1914). Section 5 dealt with prohibitions on advertising and canvassing, and in 1916 a decision was made to ensure that the 'generally recognised rules of medical ethics' were being taught in all the medical schools (General Medical Council 1916).

After the war was over new plans for health services were suggested. The Dawson Report (Dawson 1920) aimed for the establishment of health centres and the close identification of preventive and curative services. The profession had been nominally unified by the Medical Act of 1858. As we have seen there were strong pressures from GPs to make the work of consultants more easily distinguishable from their own. Dawson, however, wanted the opposite — to bring them into a more co-operative, less competitive relationship, in which referral between different types of doctor would be made easier for the benefit of patients. His health centres included space for community services, GPs consulting rooms, inpatient beds for less serious cases, and were intended to encourage consultants to attend in a visiting capacity. The idea of referral not only between individual doctors but between hospitals as treatment became more complex was finding support. However, the old anxieties were still there. Specialists, who alone were appointed to the staff of hospitals, were not prepared to let practitioners have access to the beds, and practitioners were threatened by the thought of unenviable comparisons being drawn if patients had the experience of being able to consult either a GP or a specialist in health centres. Dawson apparently never understood this, and as a result his co-operative venture did not flourish.

The technical advances in surgery and blood transfusion stimulated by the First World War, which had also produced great changes in the quality of nursing care, coupled with radiography, radiotherapy, and laboratory medicine contributed to making the 1920s a time when the stigma of hospital care was decreasing and standards were rising. GPs found that more and more of medical care seemed to be out of their reach and specialists found that where, before, hospital work was a charitable duty carried on beside their private practice, they now needed beds in properly equipped hospitals in which to treat their patients. The result was that consultants, wanting to take advantage of hospital facilities, needed to persuade paying patients of the need to enter hospitals which had previously been reserved for charity cases. In this way the question of pay-beds in voluntary hospitals became important. The questions arose of who should be able to admit patients to such beds, and whether they could be paid for providing care in institutions which had been founded as charities. If the consultant staff saw such patients gratis this meant they were losing their own livelihood. If they saw them for modest fees they undermined the GPs, who demanded the right to care for their own patients in the hospital and be paid for it, as they were in cottage hospitals. This the consultants would not concede. However, if the hospital staff charged high fees the charitable basis of the hospital was destroyed and it ceased to be able to provide for those for whom it was founded.

Practitioners, protecting their living, tried to band together to refuse referral to hospitals and specialists who were prepared to agree to work in a hybrid system where they charged hospital patients, but at below accepted consulting rates. This referral boycott failed, as had the one in 1886, at least partly because the argument over pay-beds was largely confined to London where so many of the country's consultants were concentrated. Elsewhere the problem remained that of a large population of both practitioners and patients who had no access to either specialized hospitals or consultants.

Perhaps connected with this dispute the unethical practice of fee-splitting re-emerged in the 1930s, drawing routine expressions of disapprobation from the profession's leaders. Fee-splitting was the secret agreement of the GP and specialist that, in return for the favour of the referral, the consultant would return part of the patient's fee to the GP as a commission. This required a covert relationship between GP and consultant reminiscent in some respects of that between some physicians and apothecaries in the seventeenth century. There is little doubt that this relationship exists between practitioners wherever both need to extract a living from a limited, competitive market. Because of its unethical and, in the UK, illegal nature (in UK civil law all secret commissions are declared against the public interest and illegal), it is rarely acknowledged.

A potential Pandora's box was opened by a letter in the Lancet of 4 March 1933 (Lancet 1933), written by a London surgeon who signed himself 'Unwilling Accomplice'. In this letter he claimed that he was solicited to take part in the practice of fee-splitting by at least half the practitioners who referred him patients and that unless he acquiesced he could expect to lose the majority of his practice. He identified three types of fee-splitting. The first, in which he claimed never to be involved, was the 'honest' type where GP and specialist openly agreed terms in advance of the patient's consultation. The other types, over which he felt he had no control, consisted of the GP unilaterally telling the specialist of his intention to withhold part of the patient's fee, or the specialist paying a cheque back to the practitioner. This letter drew enough attention to result in a leader in the BMJ the following week (British Medical Journal 1933), and it was apparently noticed in the national press. However, if 'Unwilling Accomplice' intended to shake the conscience of the medical world, he failed. Four letters were published on the subject in the BMJ and Lancet during the next few weeks, none of them supporting his allegations as to the extent of fee-splitting.

The GMC let it be known that the practice of fee-splitting was definitely unprofessional. The Editor of the BMJ wrote 'How far fee-splitting has become established is impossible to say. It has certainly appeared in London, but there is no evidence of its degree, or of its extension to the provinces'. But then, since it was secret, illegal, and liable to get you struck from the Register, that is hardly surprising. We shall never know whether this side-line on referral was, as 'Accomplice' stated, a routine aspect of specialist practice in the 1930s. The temptation must have been very strong.

After 40 years of the NHS it is hardly possible for us to envisage, taking the country as a whole, how few doctors in the 1930s and 1940s were engaged in full consultant practice, and consequently how many doctors had developed skills as part-time specialists but continued to practise as generalists as well. The incredulity with which we now think of the laparotomies performed in cottage hospitals by part-time GP surgeons shows how far we have ignored the realities of finance, travel, and simple availability of such recent times. Nevertheless, there was a very large gap between the expertise of many GP surgeons and the best care available from specialists, and the criticisms levelled by the leaders of the profession against GP surgeons played a significant part in the gradually dawning realization that any system of national health required attention to be paid to more than the number of doctors, their financial interests, and the quality of the best hospitals. The service could not continue to be haphazard, uncoordinated, and dominated by market forces; in short, planning was required. But making plans is no use if they can not be implemented, and thus far no significant group of doctors had been willing to accept the consequences of planning, that the service would require not only control of the number of doctors but direction of where they could work. This was a critical point; if consultants were widely distributed they would certainly provide a more comprehensive service.

However, it was not clear which doctors were going to risk their professional futures by trying to establish themselves away from the major centres of population. Thus, with planning went questions about what resources existed and how they could be distributed to allow an acceptable degree of accessibility all over the country, acceptable being judged in terms of both the doctors and the electorate.

Right up until the time when preparations for the Second World War began there were no details even of the number of hospitals in the country. Recognizing the threat of air attack as the major fear in a European war, air-raid planning began in 1935 (Dunn 1952). Recognizing also that the great London teaching hospitals would be likely to be early casualties, and needing to plan for the evacuation of great cities and the care of large numbers of injured, a comprehensive survey of hospitals was completed. An emergency medical service (EMS) was planned, and having found that it was possible to commandeer all hospitals and direct the place of work of medical staff, further efforts were made during the war to ascertain the number and distribution of specialists throughout the country. This work was carried out largely through the Nuffield Provincial Hospitals Trust, and makes sobering reading. There were probably 2800 full-time consultants in the whole country in 1938/9 (Stevens 1966). One third of these were in London. In the whole of East Anglia (Ministry of Health 1945), a region comprising Cambridgeshire, Norfolk, and Suffolk, there were only six full-time hospital obstetricians, and only four full-time psychiatrists. There was no hospital-based consultant paediatrician anywhere in East Anglia until after the end of the war. In the Oxford region (including Berkshire, Buckinghamshire, and Oxfordshire) in 1945 there were six consultant physicians, five of them based in Oxford. Two hospitals had weekly visits by consultant physicians from London. One hospital had an attached paediatrician.

Against this background of inadequate and maldistributed resources the NHS was introduced. The hospitals were nationalized at a stroke. The division of the medical profession into salaried hospital specialists, with control of the hospital beds, and self-employed GPs, excluded from hospitals but with personal registered lists which covered the whole population, was made complete. Referral lost the elements which still made it contentious. The imperative for GPs to maintain jealously-guarded lists was superseded by a payment system which involved a salary element as well as item of service payments and capitation fees, and this change was given practical expression in the abolition of the sale of the 'goodwill' of practices. Specialists had no need to accumulate private patients and, when they did so, it had ceased to be a threat to the income of the great majority of GPs. The referral system which had developed informally, and under which specialists only offered consultations to patients referred by their practitioner, and in which attendance at outpatients was also governed by the recommendation of another doctor, was transformed under the NHS into the GP's gatekeeping role. Indeed, the necessity of placing a limit on the free flow of patients from the community to specialists and hospitals was recognized from the first as being an essential part of limiting NHS costs. This at least partly explains why GPs remained fundamental to the medical system in the UK but became so much less important in the USA, where the facilitation of the rapid and frequent contact of patient and specialist constitutes such an essential part of making a professional living.

Thus, for 40 years no one has enquired too closely into referrals. By and large GPs have set their threshold for referral at a level with which specialists have coped and which patients have accepted. It was known that there was wide variation in the referral behaviour of individuals, but these were anecdotal, consisting largely of a consciousness in hospitals that particular doctors seemed to send up a lot more than their fair share of patients, and a stock of stories about referral letters consisting of requests to 'please see and advise'.

However, in the late 1980s and early 1990s the NHS has been extens- ively reviewed with the aim of ensuring greater efficiency and value for money. The relationship between those who provide services and those who make demands on services has been analysed as never before and, in that context, the decision to move a patient's care from community to hospital has been seen as both a possible surrogate measure for quality and a critical component in the consumption of resources. Stories of 25-fold variation in referral rates between practitioners have been given credence by senior politicians and, in the context of rising waiting-lists and resources overwhelmed, it is easy to seé why. Inevitably, consultants, despairing in overflowing outpatient departments and adding patients to waiting-lists from which they are destined never to be admitted, have voiced criticism of the training of practitioners and the quality of their referrals. Thus referrals have, probably rightly, become an issue again. For the first time the systematic collection of referral statistics is an obligation on all NHS GPs. The remainder of this book will guide us to understanding of what we are to make of the data.

Conclusion

Referral of patients from one doctor to another is a recent phenomenon. Conflicts between practitioners over the care of the same patient helped to define professional roles and responsibilities in the late 19th and early 20th centuries. The advent of the National Health Service quietened the remaining anxieties of the 1930s because doctors' income ceased to be dependent on whether patients consulted general practitioners or specialists. In the 1990s, the effect of the Health Service Review will be to renew interest in referral because of its variability and its potential as a surrogate measure of quality.

References

Abel Smith, B. (1964). *The hospitals 1800–1948: a study in social administration in England and Wales.* Heinemann, London.

British Medical Journal (1878). Consultants' etiquette. *British Medical Journal* **1**, 647–8.

British Medical Journal (1886*a*). Consultants and general practitioners. *British Medical Journal* **1**, 1114–5.

British Medical Journal (1886*b*). Association of general practitioners. *British Medical Journal* **1**, 1124–5.

British Medical Journal (1906). Obligations of a consultant. *British Medical Journal* **1**, 118.

British Medical Journal (1908). Central Ethical Committee: ethics of medical consultation. *British Medical Journal* **1** (Supplements), 241–3.

British Medical Journal (1910). A special class of consultants. *British Medical Journal* **1** (Supplements), 322–6.

British Medical Journal (1933). Fee-splitting. *British Medical Journal* **1**, 422.

Dawson, B. (1920). Consultative council on medical and allied services. *Interim Report*, Cmd 693. HMSO, London.

Dunn, C.L. (1952). *History of the second world war.* The emergency medical services, Vol. 1, p. 7. HMSO, London.

General Medical Council (1893). *Minutes of the Medical Council* **XXXi**.

General Medical Council (1914). *Minutes of the Medical Council* **Li**, 54–9.

General Medical Council (1916). *Minutes of the Medical Council* **Liii**, 328.

Gregory, J. (1772). *Lectures on the duties and qualifications of a physician.* London.

Kerrison, R. (1814). *An enquiry into the present state of the medical profession in England.* London.

Lancet (1933). Dichotomy. *Lancet* **1**, 493.

Loudon, I. (1986). *Medical care and the general practitioner 1750–1850.* Clarendon Press, Oxford.

Ministry of Health (1945). *The hospital services of the Eastern Area.* HMSO, London.

Stevens, R. (1966). *Medical practice in modern England: the impact of specialisation and state medicine.* Yale University Press, New Haven.

3 The interface between general practice and secondary care in Europe and North America

Douglas Fleming

Introduction — differences in health care systems

When a patient decides to consult a doctor in the UK he almost invariably sees his own GP or one of his partners. This is not the case for many other countries in the world, where long-term registration of patients with a GP is the exception rather than the rule, and where the opportunity for direct access to specialists is often available. Once contact with a primary care doctor has taken place, the doctor concerned may choose to deal with the problem himself or utilize the services of other doctors or medical workers. Again, the range of options varies greatly between countries. Thus both patient and doctor approach the consultation with prior expectations which depend on the particular health care system in which they work.

Medical care provided in different countries is also characterized by widely differing approaches to common clinical problems. As an example, 31 per cent of patients with otitis media receive antibiotics in Holland compared to 98 per cent in Australia (Froom *et al*. 1990). In Finland myringotomy is a common general practice procedure. These differences represent true differences in management approach. Other apparent differences are more concerned with preferences among alternative diagnostic labels. It is very difficult to compare national statistics concerning the incidence or prevalence of asthma, chronic bronchitis, and emphysema because the terms are used differently. In some German-speaking countries, much emphasis is placed on convalescent care and routine annual 'convalescent care holidays' are included amongst the medical benefits of insurance schemes. Such cross-national differences are not of course confined to primary care, and the examples of large differences in caesarean section rates (Notzen *et al*. 1987) and in rates for prostatectomy and hysterectomy (McPherson *et al*. 1981) between countries are well known.

In this chapter some of the differences in the ways in which patients gain access to specialist advice and treatment in different countries are described. When comparisons are made between health care systems we need to appreciate that there is in each country a unique blend of influences on decision-making processes. The European General Practice Research Workshop (Hull 1982) has undertaken two projects which have been supported by COMAC–HSR (EC Concerted Action Committee on Health Services Research) to study the differences between European health care systems. The first was concerned with the structure of primary care (COMAC–HSR 1990) and details from this study are given in the first part of the chapter. The second study involved operational research into the referral process — the European Study of Referrals from Primary to Secondary Care (COMAC–HSR 1992) — and some results from this study are described later in the chapter. Although the study was given the title 'Referrals from Primary to Secondary Care', it was concerned only with referrals from general practice care to specialist care.

In the early development of these projects it soon became apparent that the concept of primary care was viewed differently in the various countries. Confusion was increased by the term 'ambulatory care' which is applicable to all non-hospitalized persons and is therefore slightly different from 'primary care'. In the UK the term 'primary care' is closely identified with general practice, but in most European countries it is applied to all care available from a primary provider, i.e. a professional health care worker who can be approached directly without referral from some other medical or related agency. Thus, much specialist outpatient work in Europe is still within the orbit of primary care. Primary care providers may also be non-medical — for example, osteopaths, physiotherapists, and midwives. There are also difficulties in interpretation because in some countries there are two systems of primary care. In Holland and Ireland, for example, the capitation-based national health care system coexists with private insurance schemes which cover a substantial proportion of the population.

It is also relevant here to note the dynamic nature of health care delivery. In between the planning stage of the European Study of Referrals and its completion we have witnessed the virtual collapse of the primary health care system in Eastern Germany in favour of the West German equivalent. In the UK during the same period a new contract between the Department of Health and GPs as the providers of primary care has subtly influenced the relationship between GPs and patients. There is a new emphasis on the role of the GP as a provider of preventive care services delivered primarily for the benefit of the patient, but also for the GP in terms of his remuneration. In the Republic of Ireland the system of co-payments for hospital-based care has changed in a way which encourages patients towards the private sector. In Spain the development of health centres is changing the traditional pattern of health care. In Portugal recruitment to general practice has been given a national priority, so much so that 53 per cent of Portuguese GPs participating in the European Study of Referrals were aged less than 35 years (UK equivalent 33 per cent), reflecting the enormous influx of young GPs into Portuguese health care.

Health-care systems in developed countries can be considered in three main groupings (OECD 1987).

1. The National Health Service model — typified in the UK with universal coverage available for all patients and strong national control of expenditure and resources.

2. The social insurance model — typified in France and Germany where universal coverage is provided by compulsory insurance but the insurance schemes are subject to strict controls.

3. The private insurance model — typified in the USA where the patient or consumer of health care is free to take the insurance cover he considers most appropriate to his requirements and the insurance companies pay little direct part in controlling health care expenditure. This model has not been adopted in such an overt form in any European country.

All systems of health care aspire to providing access for all persons covered and have built in controls to minimize waste. Both the methods used to achieve these objectives and the degree of success achieved differ widely. Nevertheless, some common features of European health care systems can be identified. In all countries a distinction is made between hospital inpatient and outpatient care and there are often different financial arrangements for their provision, especially in countries where medical care is arranged through insurance. Until recently, control of expenditure has generally been more concerned with hospital costs than with primary care. This may be changing partly because so much can now be done without the need for hospitalization, partly because the gatekeeping role of primary care physicians is being seen as a mechanism for containing hospital costs, and partly because pharmaceuticals are largely consumed by non-hospitalized patients.

Co-payment (part payment by the patient) occurs in every health care system. In the UK, for example, co-payments are made by most people aged 16–65 years towards the cost of drugs, spectacles, and so on. In almost all countries co-payments have been introduced for pharmaceuticals, but the other services for which co-payment is expected vary greatly between countries. In countries where health care is provided through insurance schemes, the method for co-payments can have a strong influence on the system. In the USA, for example, a patient in an insurance scheme will receive a bill from a physician operating in the primary care sector, of which only a fixed amount is reimbursable through his insurance policy. The 'co-payment' is in effect negotiated between the physician and the patient. By contrast, in France the cost of the services are generally fixed and the patient settles his account and is reimbursed through his insurance.

Control of expenditure is limited in other ways: perhaps the most significant is patient registration. In the UK and Holland patient registration is usual, which effectively prevents people from shopping around at least on a large scale. In some countries — for example, Germany and Switzerland — a person can receive from his insurance scheme up to four vouchers a year which he can use to consult physicians in primary care. Here, one physician in primary care may authorize referral to another and this may include referral from what in the UK would be equivalent to a GP referring to a specialist. In some countries the voucher system for referrals is valid only for a limited period. In the European Study of Referrals 40.3 per cent of referrals in Italy were re-referrals (referral in the same specialty for the same problem within three years), a figure which is compared with 9.2 per cent in Holland and 19.0 per cent in the UK. Many of the Italian re-referrals were necessary because the authorizing referral voucher had expired. Some of the differences in the structure of primary care are illustrated by brief descriptions of health care systems in European and North American countries in the following section.

Primary and secondary care in individual countries

Austria

Health services are funded through a number of health insurance schemes which cover almost the entire population. Enhanced benefits can be obtained by making supplementary premiums. Patients are not formally registered with a GP, but a patient is tied to one doctor for the rest of that three-month period once he has consulted him for medical treatment. Many specialists work outside hospital in specialist clinics (Ambulatorien) and patients have direct access to these specialists. The work of community-based specialists, especially in cities, bears close resemblance to that of GPs, except that they do not do home visits. For laboratory work or X-ray investigations, however, a referral (from a GP or a specialist) is necessary.

Belgium

Compulsory sickness insurance covers 99 per cent of the population. Patients make a small contribution towards hospital care and primary care services are subjected to co-payments of 5–25 per cent. Specialists and GPs exist alongside each other in most parts of Belgium and the patient is free to approach either. In general, there are no financial constraints on the direct access of patients to specialists, though in some insurance schemes there are financial advantages for patients to seek specialist opinion following referral from a GP. Patients also have direct right of access to hospitals. The relationship between a patient and the doctor of his choice is freer in Belgium than in almost all other countries of Western Europe, and this liberal system has sometimes been described as a 'no system system'.

Canada

Approximately 75 per cent of health care in Canada is financed by publicly-funded schemes shared between federal and provincial governments. This is in great contrast to Canada's southern neighbour. Patients generally have a GP as first point of contact, with referral on to a specialist as necessary. In contrast to most European countries, Canadian GPs usually work in groups, often in health centres well staffed with nurses and ancillary staff. Particularly in remote rural areas, GPs may provide a substantial amount of hospital care and most Canadian GPs have hospital privileges, including admission rights and access to a wide range of sophisticated investigative facilities. In some areas there are financial incentives to encourage GPs to use community-based rather than hospital-based services for their patients.

Denmark

The entire population is covered by a compulsory insurance scheme which provides free medical care apart from co-payment for drugs. 7 per cent of the population take a higher-level insurance which gives them direct access to specialists in all branches of medicine, though they must then make a 50 per cent contribution to the cost of ambulatory care. For the majority of people, therefore, specialist care is available only after referral from the registered GP. Specialists in ophthalmology and otorhinolaryngology are exceptions to the general rule. Many of them work exclusively from their own private premises and all people have direct access to them. In other specialties, private practice exists alongside the compulsory insurance scheme with access by referral from GPs, or by direct approach for persons willing to pay or insured at the appropriate higher level.

Finland

Membership of the national insurance scheme is compulsory. Most GPs work in health centres and are salaried. There is a clear distinction between primary and secondary care, and access to hospital-based specialist treatment follows referral by the GP. Treatment in health centres is free, but there is a modest charge for hospital treatment. A small amount of specialist private practice exists, to which patients have direct access.

France

The majority of the population is covered by a compulsory national health insurance programme usually organized through employers. The benefits cover the cost of hospital treatment; but for services such as the fees of the specialists, fees in primary care, and the cost of pharmaceuticals, only partial reimbursement is made up to about 75 per cent of the total cost. Most GPs are in single-handed practice. About half the specialists work at least partly in private practice.

In the European Study of Referrals the rates of referral in France were particularly low. Patients commonly consult specialists working in an ambulatory care environment by direct approach, and patients are free to consult the specialist of their choice. Recently, as part of a series of measures to limit health care expenditure, the French government has proposed providing superior insurance cover for patients who remain registered with one primary care physician. If admission to hospital is indicated, a specific referral to a hospital-based specialist is necessary.

Germany

The state run East German system in which GPs, internists, and some-times surgeons provided primary care services from a 'Polyklinik' has been changed since German unification. Previously, access to secondary care was only by referral from a Polyklinik. Although some Polykliniks continue to operate, the whole country is moving over to the West German system where the population is covered by health insurance schemes. Patients may consult GPs or specialists. Both specialists and GPs provide primary care, though the number of community-based specialists exceeds the number of GPs, resulting in substantial competition between doctors. Many specialists work largely or exclusively in ambulatory settings, and hospital treatment is virtually limited to inpatient care. There is thus a potential referral chain from GP to outpatient specialist to inpatient specialist. Some insurance schemes offer financial advantages to patients who see specialists following referral from GPs. The system encourages very high referral demand and thus indirect referrals are commonly made. There are in effect three types of medical care: general practice based community care, specialist community or outpatient care and hospital care. There is heavy consumption of medical services both in hospital and in general practice.

Greece

Approximately 95 per cent of the population are covered by one of a number of insurance schemes. The introduction of GPs is relatively new to Greece, ambulatory care having previously been provided by community-based internal medicine specialists and paediatricians. In rural areas a substantial number of health centres have been established, increasingly staffed by GPs. These health centres provide care which is free, apart from co-payment for pharmaceuticals. In the rural areas, secondary care is generally arranged by referral from GPs. In urban areas health centres have yet to be established and patients have free access to specialists, most of whom engage in ambulatory care of one sort or another. In urban areas relatively few doctors work full time in general practice. There is intensive use of hospital outpatient departments, to which patients have direct access. Patients consulting specialists outside the hospital have to pay a variable proportion of the cost, depending on their insurance scheme.

The Republic of Ireland

For approximately 40 per cent of the population there is a national system of health care. Within this system services are provided free of charge both at primary and secondary care levels. The remaining 60 per cent of the population are responsible for their own health care costs and these are largely financed through private insurance schemes. Half of these (30 per cent of the entire population) take out enhanced insurance cover which covers them for health care costs in private hospitals and by specialists in the private sector.

Entitlement of free medical care is income related. Those on low incomes (the 40 per cent referred to above) are entitled to free medical care, including drugs. Those with middle incomes (45 per cent of the population) receive free hospital and preventive care (through their basic insurance) but must pay privately for primary non-preventive care, while those with higher incomes (15 per cent of the population) pay hospital consultant fees in addition. GPs, most frequently working single-handed, provide almost all care outside hospital settings, with a relatively small amount of specialist care available in the community, on a private basis. A tradition of specialist services provided after referral from GPs is largely observed regardless of income or insurance status. Where patients have taken out enhanced insurance there is some pressure on GPs to approve referrals automatically. Obstetric services are an exception, direct access being quite common here.

Italy

There is a National Health Service in Italy financed by taxation, although patients make a payment towards hospital consultations and investigations. An extensive system of private health care exists alongside this, and up to 50 per cent of hospital admissions in Southern Italy and 25 per cent in the North are to private hospitals. Most GPs work in single-handed practice. Specialist outpatient departments (consultori) offer direct access to ophthalmology, paediatric, dental, gynaecological, and obstetric services. For other specialties treatment is only covered by the national scheme if the patient has been referred by his or her GP. Access to these specialties therefore usually follows referral.

Netherlands

A compulsory insurance scheme covers 60 per cent of the population up to a fixed wage level. Above this level private insurance schemes operate.

An additional state-run scheme (AWBZ) covers some exceptional expenditure — for example, hospital stays exceeding one year — though recent proposals would extend the scope of the AWBZ in addition to introducing elements of competition and market forces into health care provision. GPs, who increasingly work in group practices, receive capitation fees for patients registered with them in a system more like the UK NHS than any other European country. Specialists work largely in hospitals, though some have outpatient private practices. Reimbursement for specialist care (apart from Accidents and Emergencies) is dependent on GP referral. Hospital treatment is reimbursed for up to a year after referral, following which a further referral is required.

Norway

A National Health Service covers the entire population. Hospital costs are free at the point of consumption; co-payments exist for primary care and for drugs (excepting for low-income groups). There are approximately three specialists for every two GPs. Most specialists work in hospitals, though they may have private practices in their spare time. About 5 per cent of doctors work exclusively in the private sector.

Specialist treatment is theoretically only available after referral, though in practice about 10 per cent of patients are seen without referral. When a patient is referred to hospital he is generally seen by the specialist on duty. Choice of specialist can be achieved only by referral to specialists in private practice, in which case the fees may be covered by a private insurance scheme.

Portugal

A national scheme of social security provides for health care though co-payments are necessary for some items such as drugs. Certain employment groups arrange enhanced insurance, and for these groups there is the option of direct access to specialists. Primary care is increasingly provided from health centres where GPs have personal lists of registered patients. Specialists work exclusively in hospitals, and for those with no enhanced insurance access is available only by referral from their GP.

Spain

Almost all the population is covered by the state insurance scheme INSALUD. In towns and large cities, large outpatient clinics (ambulatorio) employ specialists, GPs, and paediatricians. These cover areas of around 200 000 people. Each area has a number of smaller health care centres (consultorios) staffed by 16–18 GPs and paediatricians. Over the next few years the whole country will be covered by integrated primary health care centres (centros de salud), staffed by GPs and ambulatory specialists. The specialists will normally have their own private practice in addition.

The patient's first point of contact is with the GP who may refer him to a specialist working in an ambulatorio or to a hospital-based department. A GP may only refer to an assigned list of specialists. If the patient wishes to see another specialist then he must change his or her GP. Direct access to specialists other than paediatricians is not generally covered by INSALUD.

Sweden

There is a national health insurance scheme covering every Swedish citizen. Contributions are compulsory and are income related. Inpatient hospital care is free at the point of consumption but ambulatory care, whether specialist or generalist, involves some element of co-payment. The position of general practice in Sweden is relatively weak and there are eight times as many specialists as GPs. Most specialists work in public hospitals and patients have access to them either directly or via referral from GPs. Referrals are usually made to a specialist department rather than to a named specialist.

Switzerland

There are several health insurance sick funds and various levels of insurance. Most health service costs are covered by the schemes but varying co-payments are necessary for most services. There is a financial procedure where a patient in effect registers with a doctor for three months, and this may be a specialist or a GP, depending upon the nature of the problem presented. Both specialists and GPs work in the community, and both undertake home visits. Patients have free access to GPs, ambulatory specialists, or to hospital specialists. A doctor (GP or specialist) may refer to any hospital within his canton, except for highly specialized treatment where the patient may be referred to one of Switzerland's other 25 cantons.

USA

Health care in the USA is largely funded from private insurance schemes. The role of central government is limited to Medicare (for the elderly) and Medicaid (for those on low incomes). It is estimated that 15 per cent of Americans are not covered by any insurance. Family practice is recovering from a position of near extinction, and a small but increasing proportion of the population relate to one primary care physician. Most specialists provide primary office-based care. Although most health care is provided on a fee-for-service basis, a substantial proportion of the population is registered with a Health Maintenance Organisation (HMO). These provide full medical care for registered patients. Within the HMO, primary care may be provided by family physicians, but will also be provided by internists, paediatricians, gynaecologists, and so on. It is financially advantageous for HMOs to provide as much care as possible in an ambulatory setting, whereas for those in private practice the incentives are, if anything, the other way round.

Yugoslavia

Primary health care is arranged at a commune level. Each commune will have a major health centre in which 10–40 doctors are working. These will generally include specialists such as paediatricians, gynaecologists, school doctors, and occupational health doctors to whom the patient has a direct right of access (the larger clinics may also have other specialists). In addition, attached to the health centre there will be a number of local health stations in which three or four GPs care for a fixed group of patients. Apart from the above listed specialties, referral from a GP to a specialist service (rather than an individual specialist) is usual.

European Study of Referrals

In the second part of this chapter some of the differences between European countries are illustrated using data from the European Study of Referrals from Primary to Secondary Care. The study had four objectives:

(1) to quantify referral patterns from GPs to specialists in each participating country;

(2) to compare characteristics of doctors with high referral rates with those of doctors with low referral rates;

(3) to examine delay patterns in the referral process;

(4) to provide individual summary data for GP participants whereby they might compare their own performance within their national peer group.

The chief commitment of the volunteer GPs in each country was to record various details of 30 consecutive referrals to specialists together with consultation data during the period required to collect them. Thus for each referral the information collected included the age and sex of the patient, the problem occasioning referral, the type of referral (new or re-referral for the same problem within three years), the mode of referral (outpatient, inpatient, and so on), the urgency expressed by the doctor, the extent to which the doctor was influenced by the patient in making the referral, and the responsibility for the specialist's costs.

In a follow-up study we obtained the details of the first appointment, the date of communication from the specialist following that appointment, and the date of surgical intervention where appropriate.

There were 1548 doctors recruited from 15 European countries. In

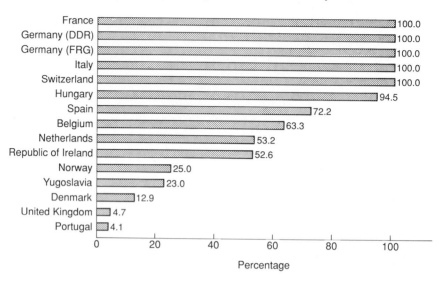

Fig. 3.1 Proportion of doctors working in solo practices.

general, they were reasonably representative by sex and age and in practice characteristics which could be compared with national data, though doctors willing to contribute to research generally are rarely representative of their peers. The total of 45 000 referrals, however, can be seen as typical of referrals made in their respective countries with regard to the study of the delay process.

Differences in practice structure

In the UK during recent years there has been an increasing tendency towards larger partnerships. To a lesser extent this tendency has occurred in Holland. In Portugal, where there is a comparatively new development of primary care based on general practice, medical groupings are very large with many groups including ten or more doctors. It is important to distinguish between doctors working together in the same premises from those which function as true partnerships. In Portugal and in Denmark many GPs share premises though do not necessarily function as a partnership at all. According to the European Study of Referrals the proportion of practitioners participating who worked alone varied from less than 5 per cent in Portugal and the UK to 100 per cent in France, Germany, Italy and Switzerland (Fig. 3.1). In general, in countries where general practice is a strong and accepted professional discipline there are more doctors working in groups. The proportion of doctors working alone is likely to

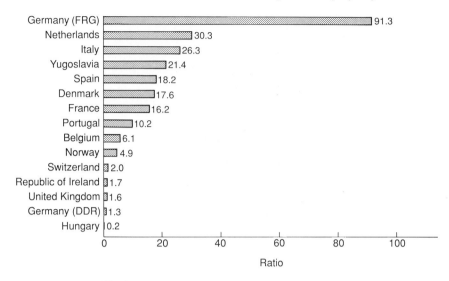

Fig. 3.2 Ratio of indirect to direct referrals (100).

decline throughout Europe, though it does not follow that doctors will necessarily work in partnership.

Indirect referrals

In the European Study of Referrals, we measured indirect referrals as well as direct referrals. An indirect referral occurs when a GP refers a patient to a specialist without an initial consultation. As an example, in the UK a child referred back to a GP by a school medical officer because of a hearing problem may be referred onward to a specialist without further assessment at a consultation. Indirect referral also occurs when a GP authorizes referral on patient demand without having first made a primary assessment. It is a condition of many insurance schemes that the GP authorizes the referral. For every 100 direct referrals recorded in the UK there were 2 indirect referrals. In West Germany there were almost as many indirect referrals as direct (Fig. 3.2). A few of the indirect referrals may have been made to extend the validity of a referral voucher and in a sense may be influenced by the specialist concerned. The majority represent consumer demand and reflect differences in patient expectations. Our colleagues in Germany work in a very competitive atmosphere. There is competition between GPs themselves and between specialists and GPs. Ready response to patient demand is the price paid by some GPs in order to keep their patients. In 1985 the cost of health care in West Germany was approximately £722 per head, twice as much as that in the UK at £364 per head (OHE 1987).

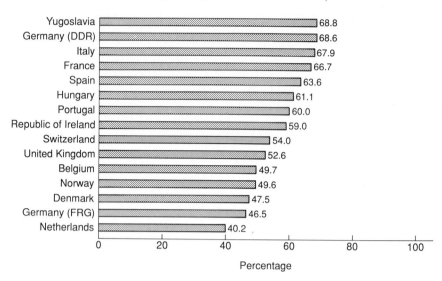

Fig. 3.3 Referrals reported with nil influence by patient.

The doctor's perception of the influence of the patient on the referral decision

For the direct referrals we examined the influence on the referral decision as perceived by the referring doctor. At each referral the doctor was asked to record whether he was influenced by the patient (nil, small, or large) in making his decision to refer. The influence in this context reflects the extent to which the doctor felt pressurized to make the referral beyond that inherent in the medical indication. The results of this analysis showed differences between countries (Fig. 3.3), which were smaller than might be expected knowing that in some countries patients have direct access to specialists independent of GPs. Roughly speaking, in most countries 20 per cent of the patients were reported to have exerted a large influence, 25 per cent a small influence, and 55 per cent nil influence. The exceptions were Holland where the respective proportions were 27 per cent large, 33 per cent small, and 40 per cent nil influence, and at the other extreme doctors in Italy expressed 12 per cent large, 20 per cent small, and 68 per cent nil influence, and the countries of Eastern Europe produced results which were similar to those for Italy. These figures tell us more about social interaction between doctor and patient than about health-care systems. Perhaps GPs in Holland more frequently see themselves as patient counsellors as opposed to health advisers. The contrast in the result for Germany as between East and West is particularly interesting since these patients had a common cultural heritage but different systems of health care.

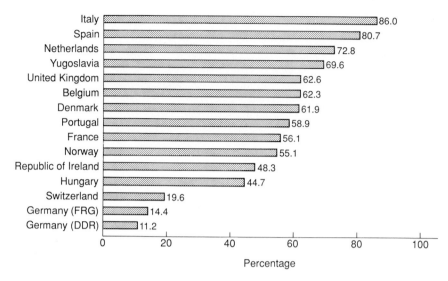

Fig. 3.4 Proportion of referrals described as routine.

Contrary to the findings reported by Armstrong *et al.* (1990) we found that the influence the patient exerted was the same among doctors who were high referrers as those who were low. For this analysis we were able to examine the referral activity of more than 1500 doctors each collecting information about 30 referrals and to standardize the data for each doctor, using the age and sex of the patients consulting and the country of origin as standardization criteria.

There were some interesting differences in the distribution of patient influence by specialty in the UK. Departures from a broadly similar pattern for most specialties occurred in dermatology, ENT, and orthopaedics, in which GPs reported substantially more pressure to refer from patients. These are three specialties where, in the UK, there are particularly long waiting-lists for hospital assessment and treatment. Unlike the situation in the UK, delays in the referral process in most other countries did not vary between specialties. There is perhaps here an inference that doctors in the UK were deliberately holding back on referrals in these specialties because they were aware of the pressures on the waiting-list, but they were nevertheless being influenced into making referrals to an extent which differed from that found in other specialties.

Urgency of referral

Recorders were asked to identify the degree of urgency (immediate, urgent, or routine). The proportion of referrals expressed as routine is given for each country in Fig. 3.4. In interpreting these figures we have to bear in mind that in some countries GPs are not so involved in emergency

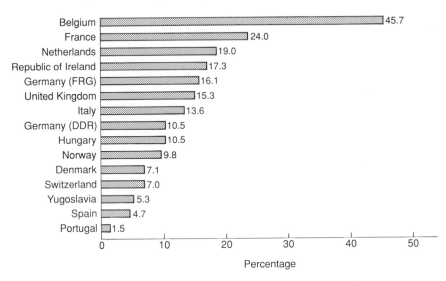

Fig. 3.5 Proportion of consultations involving a home visit.

work as in the UK, and hence the proportion of immediate referrals is artificially low. In the urban areas of Denmark and Portugal, for example, GPs are not so readily available for 24-hour cover where immediate referrals are so often necessary. Nevertheless, this comparison shows some very interesting results. In Switzerland and West Germany the majority of referrals were described as immediate or urgent. There is enormous pressure on the systems of health care in these countries to respond quickly, even though in both there were many more referrals from GPs than there were in the UK or Holland. The figures suggest that consumer-led systems such as those in Switzerland and West Germany lead to manipulation of the system to achieve objectives regardless of medical priorities. However, the availability of specialist resources may enable referring doctors to take this approach. In other countries referring doctors may be more influenced by their gatekeeping role.

In Belgium almost half (46 per cent) of all consultations take place as home visits (Fig. 3.5) and thus one would expect consumerism to be uppermost, but it is interesting to note that both in the figures for patient influence on the referral decision and for the percentage of referrals which were routine, the results for Belgium were similar to those in most other European countries.

Consultations per week

Another feature in which there were striking differences concerns the average working week of GPs (Fig. 3.6). Recorders were asked to identify the weeks during the study which should be considered as 'normal' (not

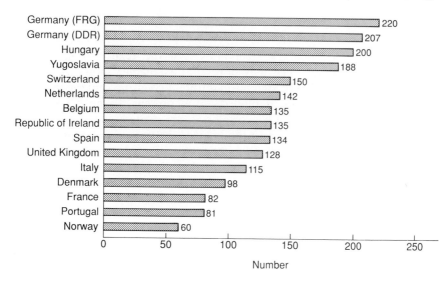

Fig. 3.6 Number of consultations in an average working week.

interrupted by personal or partnership sickness or holiday) and these were averaged for each doctor. In interpreting these data, however, we must bear in mind that the average frequency of consultation varies between countries. In Switzerland, for example, there are between seven and eight consultations per patient per annum, which is twice that in the UK. Each country has developed its own pattern of care though we cannot argue that any one pattern is based on good scientific principles. The same can be said for the relative balance of work between GPs and specialists. The issues are complex and it is difficult to draw firm conclusions without considering the content of consultations in more detail, and without considering other health care facilities available in the different countries.

Conclusion

The health care systems described in this chapter show clearly how a range of methods of providing primary care have developed. Although beyond the scope of this book, one of the important influences on the future development of relationships between GPs and specialists is the partial standardization of medical training in the EC. General practice has been developing an academic base and a specific training in many European countries over the past 20 years. The acceptance of a mandatory training period for general practice will strengthen the discipline within the EC, and it is likely that GPs across Europe will have a more coherent view of what their job involves than they do now. This is particularly likely to be the case for preventive care and long-term management of chronic disease, which are becoming increasingly important parts of general practice.

However, even though a clearer view of the relative roles of the generalist and the specialist may develop, this chapter shows that structural aspects of health care systems in different countries and the different ways in which health care is funded are at present the most important determinants of the ways in which referrals are made between generalists and specialists. Any changes to the balance of care provided in primary and secondary care in an individual country will need to involve changes both to the training of doctors and to the administrative and financial arrangements which influence referral behaviour.

Acknowledgements

The information presented in this chapter stems largely from two European co-operative studies, the Interface Study and the Study of Referrals from Primary to Secondary Care. These studies were designed in the European General Practice Research Workshop and have been financed chiefly as concerted actions sponsored by the Health Services Research Committee of the EEC. The results from the latter study which are included in this paper are based on interim analyses of the data and may be subject to small alterations in the final report.

References

Armstrong, D., Fry, J., and Armstrong, P. (1991). Doctors' perceptions of pressure from patients for referral. *British Medical Journal* **302**, 1186–8.

COMAC–HSR in collaboration with European General Practice Research Workshop (1990). *The Interface Study* (ed. D.L. Crombie, J. Van der Zee, and P. Backer), Occasional Paper No. 48, Royal College of General Practitioners, London.

COMAC–HSR in collaboration with European General Practice Research Workshop (1992). *The European Study of Referrals from Primary to Secondary Care* (project leader D.M. Fleming), Occasional Paper No. 56, Royal College of General Practitioners, London.

Froom, J., Culpepper, L., Grob, P., Bartelds, A., Bowers, P., Bridges-Webb, C., Grava-Gubins, I., Green, L., Lion, J., Somaini, B., Stroobant, A., West, R., and Yodfat, Y. (1990). Diagnosis and antibiotic treatment of acute otitis media: report from International Primary Care Network. *British Medical Journal* **300**, 582–6.

Hull, F.M. (1982). The European General Practice Research Workshop, 1971–1981. *Journal of the Royal College of General Practitioners* **32**, 106–8.

McPherson, K., Strong, P.M., Epstein, A., and Jones, L. (1981). Regional variations in the use of common surgical procedures: within and between England and Wales, Canada and the United States of America. *Social Science and Medicine* **15A**, 273–88.

Notzen, F.C., Placek, P., and Taffel, S.M. (1987). Comparisons of national caesarean-section rates. *New England Journal of Medicine* **316(7)**, 386–9.

Office of Health Economics (1987). *Compendium of Health Statistics*, (6th edn). OHE, London.

Organisation of Economic Cooperation and Development (1987). *Financing and Delivering Health Care*. OECD, Paris.

World Health Organisation (1985). *Targets for Health for all by 2000. Targets in support of the European Regional Strategy for Health for All*. WHO Regional Office for Europe, Copenhagen.

4 The NHS Review, 1988–1991: GPs and contracts for care

Barry Tennison

Introduction

This chapter examines the 1991 changes to the NHS and their influence on the role of GPs and the referral process. The chapter gives an outline of the NHS Review changes, describes some project work which anticipated the effects and also the early experience of the NHS internal market, and draws attention to a number of problematic areas.

Background

The NHS Review

During 1988 the UK government carried out a Review of the NHS. This led to the publication of the white paper 'Working for Patients' in January 1989 (Department of Health 1989a). Around the same time the thinking on community care was crystallized into another white paper, 'Caring in the Community' (Department of Health 1989b). These two threads gave rise to new legislation, the NHS and Community Care Act of June 1990. This was largely an enabling Act, changing the constitution of HAs and FHSAs, (the former Family Practitioner Committees), and allowing the Secretary of State for Health to make wide-ranging regulations. It also made FHSAs, like DHAs, accountable to RHAs.

The fundamental new feature of the post-Review NHS is the split between purchasers and providers of health care, and the encapsulation of the relationship between them into NHS contracts. These are a form of contract or agreement covering the quality, quantity, and price of health care services to be provided, but they are not enforceable through the courts as they are technically agreements between one part of the NHS and another. This split is reinforced by a change in the method of funding to a system of weighted capitation based on resident population, that is on people and health need, rather than on services historically provided in the locality.

This form of running of the NHS took effect on 1st April 1991. Tables 4.1 and 4.2 look further at the purchaser and provider roles.

Table 4.1 *Purchasers of health care*

1. District Health Authorities (DHAs) — have responsibility for assessing the health needs of their resident population and purchasing health care to meet these needs, within their allocated resources.

2. General Practice Fundholders (GPFHs) — purchase outpatient referrals and elective care for a specific range of conditions, mainly surgical procedures.

3. Regional Health Authorities (RHAs) — may purchase some specialised care.

4. Family Health Services Authorities (FHSAs) — may be regarded as purchasers of much primary care.

Table 4.2 *Providers of health care*

1. NHS Directly Managed Units (DMUs) — hospitals, mental health and community units of management that are under direct DHA control; these provide secondary and some primary care under NHS contracts, usually with many purchasers.

2. NHS Trusts (NHSTs) — former DMUs which have taken a new status within the NHS, independent of any DHA, and with more managerial freedom.

3. Independent sector hospitals and other providers.

4. General Practitioners — are providers of much primary care.

The role of the FHSA

The 1990 Act changed the position of the bodies administering the GP contract. Previously, FPCs had been directly accountable to central government (the Department of Health). Since September 1990 the newly constituted FHSAs have been responsible to RHAs, bringing them into a similar position to DHAs. In particular, RHAs now allocate resources to FHSAs and review their performance. RHAs are thus able to take an overview of both primary and secondary care in their geographical area, and to encourage and promote joint working and joint purchasing between DHAs and FHSAs.

Allocation of resources

A change has begun in the way in which resources are allocated to RHAs, and thence to DHAs. There is a rapid move towards a position where resources are allocated by a formula known as weighted capitation. The amount of revenue allocated depends mainly on the resident population of the RHA or DHA. This raw population figure is weighted to take account of the age distribution of the resident population (and the differing costs of health care delivery to people of different ages), and a number of other factors, including local mortality rates and social deprivation. In the short term there is also a weighting in acknowledgement of some of the special problems of the Thames Regions with regard to London.

At present resources are being allocated to GPFHs on the basis of their past patterns of care, including referrals to hospital. This money comes from RHA allocations and is deducted from the allocation of the corresponding DHA(s).

Community care

The 1990 Act also introduced a major reform in community care. Local authorities are to become the lead agency, with the obligation to produce community care plans for certain client groups (including the elderly, the mentally and physically handicapped, and the mentally ill), and to introduce care managers for individuals. The plans must include the assessment of the needs of individuals, and the purchasing of packages of care to meet the needs, from a variety of agencies, possibly including the NHS. In recognition of the substantial nature of this change and its implications, full implementation has been postponed from the originally intended date of 1st April 1991.

Local authorities are being encouraged into a purchaser role for community care services, and to reduce their activities as providers.

Early experience of policy implementation

Development projects

The time allowed for such a major reorientation of the organization of the NHS was not great. The government explicitly eschewed the idea of trials or pilots of the Review ideas and structures. However, the policies did need some development, and this was carried out partly by encouraging local projects to work on aspects of implementing the changes. These included particularly the purchaser role, provider pricing, the contractual relationship, and quality measures.

One of the main projects was the East Anglian Internal Market Project (1989–1991). Three adjacent DHAs initially experimented with NHS contracts for patients crossing district boundaries, and four other DHAs with contracts for home units (those managed by the purchasing DHA). Later, the scope was extended to include treatments of East Anglian RHA residents in any of the eight DHAs in the Region. Other projects concerning NHS contracts were carried out in the South Western RHA, and in the Yorkshire RHA for regional specialties, continuing work started before 'Working for Patients'.

Table 4.3 *DHA purchasers and GPs*

---

1. GPs control referral patterns.

2. DHAs must consult local GPs about referral preferences and opinions about quality.

3. Pressure on particular contracts can require co-operation between DHAs and local GPs.

The main focus of these projects was inpatient and day-case care, which was seen as the most important area to clarify in the light of the large proportion of NHS spending consumed in this way. (The omission of outpatient care was at least partly because of the small amount and poor quality of the available relevant information.) There was essentially no project work on GP fundholding in advance of its implementation in April 1991.

The purchaser role of DHAs and relationship with GPs

The role of the DHA purchaser involves assessment of health need; the selection of providers to meet this need; the negotiation, administration, and monitoring of NHS contracts; representation of and communication with the local population; and management of directly managed provider units. This role required substantial development, particularly in the areas of management and organization, and in the development of information and information systems for assessment of need and contract management and monitoring.

It was realized very early that, for a DHA purchaser, the role of local GPs was crucial. The DHA could set contracts with providers, but the GPs with whom their residents were registered were the people who would determine whether referrals were made in line with the contracts. Accordingly, DHAs in the Internal Market Project consulted their GPs early in the process of needs assessment and provider selection. Their views were sought by practice visits, through local GP forums, and in writing. They were asked about their opinions on local needs, about how satisfactory they found local and other providers, and about their referral practice. In many places GPs were content with local services, subject to some specific complaints, and said they sometimes referred patients to distant Units, but generally could not quantify the numbers so referred, nor the frequency.

DHAs also needed to work with GPs during the currency of the project contracts. There were some efforts to ensure that GPs continued to be willing to make their referrals in line with established contracts. In some cases, where the actual referrals turned out (in mid-contract) to

Table 4.4 *Pricing of treatments in provider units*

---

1. Pricing must be based on costs.

2. Pricing is very difficult using traditional NHS accounting methods.

3. Pricing will be harder for outpatient and ambulatory treatments than for inpatient treatment.

4. Pricing is more difficult for GPFH contracts.

---

be significantly greater than had been expected, referrals had to be discouraged. In at least one situation, this led a DHA to request that only emergency cases should be sent to a particular Unit. At contract renewal, DHAs were able to consult GPs about previous contracts, and seek their opinions about the future contracts needed.

Provider pricing

The projects tested the providers' ability to price individual inpatient stays and day-case episodes, in terms either of the specialty of treatment or of a more detailed categorization, such as operative procedure. The rules promulgated by the NHS Management Executive and the Department of Health made it clear that, for NHS Units (including NHSTs), price should equal cost, so that there should be no speculative pricing nor cross-subsidization. The use of traditional hospital (and other unit) accounting categories to assign costs to particular individual treatments or types of care is far from straightforward. The project experience suggested that available data, procedures, and expertise did allow hospitals to price inpatient stays; however, the prices derived showed a very wide variation between hospitals, reflecting the difficulty of the process. Probable explanations included errors, lack of the necessary skills, poor information systems, variation in procedures to allocate costs to stays (for example, the fixed and semi-fixed costs of overheads and of employing staff), differences in case mix, and true differences in cost.

Many units were willing to expend substantial effort on detailed pricing of stays which they felt were important to their viability in the 'market' for health care. However, no unit felt comfortable with the idea of calculating individual prices for the range of over 100 procedures covered by GP fundholding. However, as the real internal market started after April 1991 they had to do this, however crudely.

One of the features revealed by the project concerned long-stay patients, that is those patients whose planned or unplanned inpatient stay exceeded about four weeks. This category included a range of elderly or mentally ill people. Whereas units were willing to price the treatments of acute inpatients on the basis of a price per stay (technically, per consultant episode), for long-stay patients it was felt that a price per inpatient day was more appropriate after an initial period of say 28 days. When priced according to cost, these patients contributed a very substantial amount to the contractual financial commitment of DHAs.

Although not covered by the development projects, the establishment of costs (and so prices) for outpatient treatments was seen as a substantial issue. Outpatient attendances occur in very much larger numbers than inpatient and day-case treatments. They are very much more difficult to distinguish in terms of the extent to which they use hospital resources. The development of classifications of outpatient (probably to be called ambulatory) treatments and attendances, and the assignment of prices, will be a major challenge for future years.

From project to reality

At the end of the East Anglian Internal Market Project the lessons and experience were used to determine the way the Region began the real internal market after April 1991. Whereas elsewhere in England the majority of contracts were of 'block' form (that is giving a provider a fixed payment whatever the amount of contract work performed), in East Anglia the majority were in 'cost and volume' form, where the payment depends on the amount of work. Providers had had some experience of pricing treatments.

New factors in the real as opposed to the project market included payments for outpatient and community work and the introduction of GP fundholders.

Problematic areas

In the light of the early experience with the NHS Review changes there would seem to be a variety of problematic areas connected with the process of GP referral. Many of these will require some evolution of the contracting process.

The implicit view of medical practice

The majority of thinking behind the contracting process seems to be based on a very simplified view of referral practice, summarized in the sequence in Table 4.5.

This is a possible paradigm for a straightforward problem requiring elective surgery. It ignores the complicating factors that many of the problems for which GPs seek secondary advice and care are medical rather than surgical, and that around 50 per cent of admissions to hospital are as emergencies rather than from a waiting-list. More subtle forms of contract will be needed to provide useful incentives for high quality in the care of people with chronic illnesses, such as diabetes or schizophrenia.

Table 4.5 *A very simple view of the referral process*

GP consultation

→ outpatient attendance

→ waiting list

→ inpatient stay

→ follow up outpatient attendance

→ return to care of GP.

The simplistic view of the interaction between primary and secondary care also seems to carry the impression that GPs demand and obtain specific specialist services for their patients; in fact, a GP often refers with a problem, not a solution. In this case it may not be clear at the time of referral exactly which contract (or which part of the contract) a patient should fall under.

Provider services and contracting method

The variety of provider services demands a variety of modes of contracting: acute inpatients, long-stay inpatients, respite care, day cases, day care, outpatients, community services, mental health, mental handicap. It may be desirable to contract in different terms for different services. As an example, for care by community psychiatric nurses, a contract may be best phrased in terms of the number of chronically ill patients given continuing attention to specified quality standards, whereas for respite-care the number of bed days may be the best measure.

Only in some of these contexts are specialty of care and consultant responsibility important factors. For inpatient care, consultant episode or (less commonly) inpatient day may be the best contracting currency. (A consultant episode is a continuous period of inpatient treatment under the responsibility of one particular consultant.) For outpatient care it may be the attendance; however, there would be virtue in contracting for a 'course' of outpatient care, were it possible to define this with sufficient precision in a particular context. It is unclear what the optimal contracting method is, for example, for health visitor care.

Assessing and meeting health needs; DHAs and GPs

A DHA has explicit responsibility for assessing the health needs of its resident population and meeting those needs, within available resources, through NHS contracts. Meeting the health needs of a geographically defined population requires concerted action from a wide variety of individuals and organizations: GPs, health care providers, local authorities, voluntary and private organizations, individuals and their carers. These parties also have views, often differing, on what the health needs are. DHAs clearly must consult widely on the assessment of need, while bringing a population perspective to the process.

The need for DHAs to consult and inform GPs has revealed the poverty of mechanisms for doing so. Independent-minded GPs tend to be impatient with the apparently bureaucratic processes of large organizations. There is an incentive for DHAs and FHSAs to work more closely together; for example, over the assessment of need, and the incorporation of the general practice view into this. This may have the very beneficial effect of moving towards an integration of primary and secondary care, which in the UK system are organizationally separated in an uncomfortable way (NHS Management Executive 1991).

The existence of GP fundholders complicates the DHA responsibility for meeting need. GPFH budgets are funded by reducing DHA budgets. In theory, the DHA is held responsible for balancing priorities and meeting needs, even though GPFH decision-making is outside its control. Traditionally, DHAs take a population view (informed by public health expertise), while GPs take a more individually-based view. It remains to be seen whether an expansion of GP fundholding will distort the priorities for health care spending on resident populations.

GP compliance with DHA contracts

DHAs are responsible for meeting health needs through NHS contracts. A DHA's portfolio of NHS contracts will be the collection it feels are required to best meet the needs. However, it is not clear what power the DHA has to ensure that the contracts are adhered to. GPs are the people who determine actual referrals, but are not parties to NHS contracts between DHAs and provider units.

This separation of roles would appear to conflict with the traditional GP freedom of referral. A DHA will attempt to minimize GP disagreement with the portfolio of contracts by consulting over the assessment of need. However, GP opinion is quite variable, and few GPs will allow that any body can speak for them. On the other hand, a potential 'restriction' on freedom of referral is not as new as it seems. The hospital sector has in the past controlled GP referrals by rationing resources (as evidenced by waiting-lists), and even in certain cases by explicitly declining to fund treatments (for example, in the private sector, or for some very expensive treatments such as secure care of people with disturbed behaviour).

The mechanism for allowing GPs, in exceptional cases, to refer outside contracts is the so-called extracontractual referral (ECR). Since this is a potentially uncontrolled commitment to expenditure, DHAs (and the NHS Management Executive) have been at pains to minimize its occurrence. ECRs are divided into emergency and elective types. DHAs are committed to pay for emergency ECRs. However, elective ECRs should only take place with the knowledge and blessing of the responsible DHA. These include elective tertiary referrals. For elective ECRs by GPs, DHA blessing might be sought either by the referring GP, or by the unit receiving the referral. The latter has the greater incentive, since the DHA is not committed to pay if blessing has not been granted. In fact, according to current rules, it is the unit's responsibility to check with the DHA of residence before giving elective treatment; some DHAs are encouraging GPs to give them advance warning of ECRs so that they may anticipate the commitment to expenditure. Many people are concerned that patients should not become aware of any conflict over responsibility for payment for their treatment. Some authorities believe that the distinction between elective and emergency referrals is not as absolute as some might think, and anticipate a tendency to reclassify referrals as emergencies. DHAs are monitoring this.

It is of interest that in the USA, health maintenance organizations (HMOs) usually require that their permission be granted before one of their subscribers receives hospital treatment. This permission is sought by contacting a department in the HMO, often run by trained nurses. They require details of the treatments contemplated, and will usually check that they adhere to a predetermined protocol. Disputes may be referred to medical advisors. A further trend is towards third-party vetting organizations which take over this approval of care plans from the HMO.

The early experience since April 1991 suggests that there are no substantial problems over GP compliance with DHA contracts. GPs have been used to accepting the existence of waiting-lists for secondary care, and this is still the main way in which a restriction to a contracted level of activity makes itself shown. It does appear, however, that waiting-times and lengths of waiting-lists have increased in the early months after April 1991, and this is likely to lead to dissatisfaction with the NHS among the public as well as among GPs.

GP fundholding

The GP fundholder's budget covers a certain precisely defined range of hospital treatments, including the associated investigations and follow-ups. This means that hospitals' NHS contracts with GPFHs have to be more complex than those with DHAs, which (at present) separate outpatient and inpatient care. As an example, the price for a GPFH referral must include an element to cover the uncertainty about how many outpatient attendances will be needed; or alternatively, the form of pricing must avoid this uncertainty, say by charging separately for each attendance.

This, together with the fact that, initially at least, only a small proportion of most hospitals' work is GPFH funded, has led to some reluctance on the part of provider units to go to the considerable effort of quoting detailed prices for GPFH work and of negotiating NHS contracts with GPFHs. Provider units are finding it difficult to run contracts of these differing natures.

GPFHs feel that their 'purchasing power' will oblige units to satisfy them; for example, by improving quality. This may have some force where GPFHs have substantial choice in their selection of provider, as in some metropolitan districts, and where many GPs have become GPFHs. However, where this choice is small (taking into account patient preferences, for example, for local treatment), the GPFH will have less leverage. The 'provider market' aspect of the post-Review NHS is seen by its protagonists as powerful mechanism to improve quality, by the exercise of choice by DHAs and GPFHs; however, some feel that this is an ideology based on a geographical area with a relative overprovision of potentially competing hospitals, such as London.

In addition, GPFHs are finding that, whereas it may be a straight-forward matter to specify high quality in their contracts with providers, it is another matter to ensure that these are adhered to. Monitoring waiting-times, or the quality of the experience of hospital attendence, requires systematic effort. The major threat in the case of non-compliance is making referrals elsewhere, which both GPs and patients may not wish to happen, for reasons of tradition, loyalty, geography, and lack of definitely better alternatives. On the other hand, hospital consultants are, in some cases, more open to persuasion by their GP colleagues towards change than they have been to persuasion by general managers; thus GPFHs may be able to achieve improvement where managers have not, if this improvement is based on changed consultant practices.

The specification of different quality standards by different purchasers has led to accusations of two-tier care, or inequalities in the care received by patients according to the referrer. A particularly pointed case is the prospect of differential waiting-times, with the possibility of separate waiting-lists for GPFH-funded patients and DHA-funded patients. This apparent breach of the principle of treatment according to clinical need has led the NHS Management Executive to formulate rules about the way hospitals should maintain waiting-lists, designed to ensure that patients are treated according to clinical priority. While reassuring many people, this is a marked constraint on the GPFH's ability to negotiate an improved standard of care.

Different general practices have seen different reasons for becoming GPFHs. Some have done so because they felt it was essential in order to preserve their freedom of referral. Others have wished to take advantage of the substantial funding offered to improve the quality of practice management. Others have seen a benefit in being able to work with some freedom within an explicit budget, giving the opportunity to redirect financing, for example, away from hospital care and into treatments provided nearer the patient's home.

GPFH budgets (per list patient) have been markedly variable around the country, as they have so far been based on the costs of past referral patterns. It is very likely that over the next few years there will be a move towards more equitable funding, closer to the weighted capitation formula for DHAs. In this case some GPFHs, at least, may begin to feel that the funding they receive for hospital referral is inadequate. Since the funds for GPFHs are deducted from DHA budgets, and since DHAs must fund emergency care, over which they have little control, an increase in the number of GPFHs leads to a marked reduction in the freedom of manoeuvre that DHAs have to remain within budget without curtailing essential care. This factor alone will be a pressure towards the rationalization of the size of GPFH budgets.

In some areas GPFHs have seen the advantages of coming together into larger groups, to enhance their negotiating position and to share the burden of contract negotiation and management. Further, they might share the process of needs assessment, which is the foundation on which contracted amounts of care should be based, and in many places GPFHs are seeing the advantage of sharing this task with the local DHA. Alternatively, groups of GPFHs could be seen to be effectively beginning to reconstitute an HA, and this might happen particularly where GPs have been dissatisfied with their local DHA.

The existence of GPFHs means that the NHS internal market, always intended to have competing providers, also has competing purchasers. A patient might choose to register with a GPFH rather than a non-GPFH because in the latter case it would be a DHA's contracts which would apply. Internationally, health systems with competing purchasers show marked inefficiency, with high administrative costs; this applies to most insurance-based systems, such as those in France, Germany, and the USA.

Table 4.6 summarizes some of the advantages and disadvantages of GP fundholding.

Caring in the community

A major potential conflict lies in the distinction between 'health care' and 'social care'. Over the next 20 years the number of elderly people requiring community care is set to rise substantially. In addition, people with chronic mental illnesses and mental handicap are being moved out of institutional care. 'Caring in the Community' gives local authorities the lead responsibility for co-ordinating community care, but HAs have responsibility for purchasing that component deemed to be health care. The boundary between health care and social care is very grey. As an example, a person with dementia often requires attention of a nursing kind — for example, to prevent pressure sores — but not for a strict medical indication, and the person with chronic mental illness also may need persuasion to keep taking their medication.

Table 4.6 *Some advantages and disadvantages of GP fundholding*

Advantages

1. GP has more choice and freedom.

2. GP has incentive to find most cost effective care.

3. GP and patient may be treated better by providers.

4. Contracts with GPFH give incentive to providers to improve quality.

Disadvantages

1. Decisions may be made on financial rather than clinical grounds.

2. Having competing purchasers leads to inefficiency and inequity.

3. Greater complexity of administration and management, particularly for GPFHs and providers.

4. DHAs are less able to fulfil their role of fulfilling the health needs of their resident population.

The proposals envisage the appointment of care managers who will be responsible for constructing care plans and commissioning the required care, following the assessment of individual needs. In the future GPs will probably find themselves making ('social') referrals to these care managers.

Information

The operation of the post-Review NHS requires a substantial enhancement of NHS information and information flows. As an example, data must pass from provider to purchaser to justify payment for treatments carried out, purchasers need enhanced information support for assessing health needs, and information will be needed to monitor the operation of the market.

Purchasers (DHA or GPFH) require data about treatments delivered to their residents (or, for GPFHs, their registered patients), both to monitor contracts and ECRs and to contribute to their knowledge of health need. Information is required on all categories of treatment: inpatients, day-cases, outpatients, accident and emergency, respite care, long stay, community services, and others. In a substantial number of these contexts a contract minimum data set has been devised, containing the minimum amount of information a purchaser requires from a provider for each treatment. Within contract negotiation, agreement can be reached that more data should be provided beyond this minimum. Progress with outpatient and community minimum data sets is planned over the years to 1993/4, as these are less well developed.

The present minimum data sets do not contain any reference to prices or costs. Most purchasers will wish to receive price information for each chargeable episode or treatment. In addition, the minimum data sets and supplementary information will be the means by which purchasers will monitor case mix and effectiveness, using outcome measures. GPFHs may be unfamiliar with the use of minimum data sets and may not particularly wish to receive them. However, providers expect to send minimum data sets with all invoices for payment under NHS contracts.

A standard referral letter data set has been devised. This is required to enable a provider to determine the responsible purchaser (DHA or GPFH) and the relevant contract. It includes patient details, such as NHS number, name, and address (including postcode), and details of referral, including consultant and specialty. In future, GPs will be expected to use a standard form of referral, including this data as a minimum. This data set will need to be introduced sensitively, and it may need modification and development.

So that DHAs can fulfil their function of monitoring their residents' health and assessing their needs, NHS provider units will send to the relevant DHA a copy of the contract minimum data set for any GPFH-funded treatment. At present, treatments entirely in the independent sector do not give rise to any such passing of data.

GPFHs are expected to find that they need substantially enhanced information systems to fulfil their new role. In addition to contract administration and accounting, they should investigate and assess their patients' needs for the treatments covered by fundholding.

Conclusion

Despite its many suggestive features, the 'market' for NHS health care is not a free market but a heavily managed one. As the changes resulting from the Review have been specified more precisely in the process of implementation, they have been subjected to more and more qualifications and rules. While this may mean that some of the potentially beneficial effects of a market place are lost, it may also be that the strong regulation manages to avert many potentially damaging consequences.

One of the declared aims of the changes was the enhancement of patient choice. However, the consumer view has not yet found an effective place. Community Health Councils continue to exist and to have a specified watchdog role, but they are mostly suspicious of the changes. Moreover, their traditional role involved monitoring providers, although they relate to Authorities who are now purchasers. DHAs, FHSAs, and GPFHs have yet to identify and implement mechanisms to incorporate the consumer view effectively.

GPs are key players in the post-Review NHS. They fulfil a variety of roles. As gatekeepers to secondary care they stand between purchasers and providers. They act as patient representatives, making or strongly influencing choices such as referral preference. They are themselves providers of primary care, effectively purchased by FHSAs. If GPFHs, they act as purchasers of certain types of care. Whether fundholders or not, they can provide a strong drive towards increased quality.

There is a potential conflict between the GP's inclination to act as an advocate for the individual patient and the view a DHA has to take of the needs of the resident population as a whole. DHAs may need to improve GP's appreciation of the requirement to balance or trade-off between options; for example, should resources be used to increase the number of cataract removals, the number of hip replacements, or the long-term care facilities for the elderly or mentally ill? Planning of capital developments, consultant and junior doctor recruitment, and the negotiation of NHS contracts require views to be taken on matters such as these, rather than on the immediate needs of individual patients.

The existence of GPFHs adds a new dimension to the NHS. Their role is not totally clear, and many uncertainties surround their participation in the internal market. This is leading to constraints being put on their freedom; for example, to negotiate NHS contracts which give their patients substantial advantages over other patients. If more GPs take up fund-holding status, the room that DHAs have to manage within tight budgets will be reduced, as they are compelled to fund emergency care.

Given that the NHS health care market is not a free one, monitoring and regulating the market is a natural role for RHAs. With their responsibility for FHSAs, GPFHs, and DHAs, they can take a global view of primary and secondary care, and assist in bringing FHSAs and DHAs closer; for example, into joint assessment of needs and joint working in purchasing. RHAs can take a strategic view on possible organizational realignments, including mergers. RHAs are to be held accountable by the NHS Management Executive and the Department of Health for delivering the NHS Review changes in effective and beneficial ways.

A marked potential benefit of the NHS Review changes is that it can make explicit the nature, quantity, and quality of the health care delivered by the NHS. This will reveal the rationing choices which have to be made, and are being made, in health care.

Referral by GPs to secondary care is a key part of the process by which health care is delivered in the UK. The NHS Review changes re-emphasize its central importance.

References

Department of Health (1989*a*). *Working for patients*. HMSO, London.
Department of Health (1989*b*). *Caring in the community*. HMSO, London.
NHS Management Executive (1991). *Integrating primary and secondary health care*, reference EL (91) 27. Department of Health.

5 Measuring referral rates

Martin Roland

Introduction

At the time that the government published its White Paper on primary health care in the UK in 1987 a number of research studies, reviewed in Chapter 6, had suggested that there was wide variation among GPs in their rates of referral to hospital. This variation was interpreted by the Department of Health (1987) as indicating inefficient use of resources:

Health Authorities incur a very substantial cost through family doctors' decisions to refer patients to hospital and through their use of hospital diagnostic and treatment facilities. It is important that expensive hospital facilities are used in the most cost effective way, and the wide variation in referral rates suggests that this may not always be the case. Family doctors (who have no information about costs) have little reason to examine their criteria for referral. While in some circumstances, a higher than average referral rate may be justified, a minority may refer substantially more patients to hospital than the requirements of the individuals concerned merit. Patients whose doctors make fewer than average referrals may not benefit fully from the hospital facilities available for their conditions.

Until that time there had been no systematic way of recording the number of patients sent to hospital by any one doctor or group of doctors. In 1990 and 1991 two government initiatives led to the routine collection of data on the use of hospital services by GPs, namely the requirement of GPs from April 1991 to produce an annual report containing data on their referrals, and the requirement of hospitals to collect a routine set of data on referrals, including the referring doctors, from April 1991. The type of information which will be available from these two sources is described in the first section of this chapter, before a discussion of how the data on numbers of referrals may be used to calculate referral rates to allow the behaviour of different doctors to be compared.

Counting referrals

The 1990 General Practitioner contract made specific requirements about the data to be collected regarding referral patterns. These were that the numbers of inpatient and outpatient referrals should be counted for 15 specialities, namely general surgery, general medicine, orthopaedics, rheumatology, ENT, gynaecology, obstetrics, paediatrics, ophthalmology, psychiatry, geriatrics, dermatology, neurology, genito-urinary medicine, and others. In addition, doctors were required to count referrals to X-ray departments and for pathology tests. Self-referrals were to be included 'where known'. Doctors in partnership were given the option of providing these data as individuals or as a practice.

Certainly at the start of 1990 most practices did not have in place data collection systems to count the number of referrals made to hospital. The initial quality of the data was very variable, and it is likely that there was substantial under-reporting of referrals in some practices. The quality of the data is likely to improve, though there is little incentive, financial or otherwise, for doctors to develop systems which will ensure accurate data collection of this type, and few practices currently collect routine clinical data on computer. For many practices, the secretary responsible for typing letters will be the most appropriate member of the practice team to collate referral data. One of the particular difficulties which practices are likely to experience is to ensure completeness of data collection for referrals made out of hours, for those made by deputies or locums, and for those which are made by phone or with a handwritten letter.

Apart from the quality of the data, the most serious flaw in the data required by the 1990 GP contract is that it did not include numbers of private referrals. It is known that GPs vary widely in the proportion of patients referred outside the NHS. In one study the proportion of patients referred privately varied from 4–53 per cent (Coulter *et al.* 1991). If these differences are widespread, as they are likely to be, an apparent difference in referral rates of a factor of two, judged solely by NHS referral rates, could simply be due to a failure to include private referrals. Many FHSAs have realized this, and have requested details of private referrals in GPs Annual Reports in order to make their data more meaningful in future years.

The routine collection of referral data by hospitals is potentially a more reliable method of data collection than using data from practices, and from April 1991 a set of data to be collected on each referral was specified by the government. This minimum data set included information on both the referring doctor and the doctor with whom the patient was registered. Although this system may become the method of choice for collecting referral data for some purposes — for example, for setting purchasing contracts — it has serious drawbacks as far as comparing GPs' referral behaviour is concerned. The first drawback is the absence of information on private referrals. These data can be requested from GPs in their Annual Reports, but they cannot be provided by a hospital-based data collection system unless private hospitals are included, which is unlikely in the near future. The second major problem of data collection by hospitals is collation of data from several hospitals or HA areas. In a study in the Oxford Region, GPs referred to an average of 16 hospitals (Coulter *et al.* 1989), and the number may be considerably greater in metropolitan areas. Collation of data from different hospitals is being piloted in the East

Anglian region, and it may be possible to aggregate data from all the hospitals in this region from April 1991. The system would give valuable information about the referral patterns of East Anglian GPs, as extra regional referrals account for less than 3 per cent of referrals in East Anglia. However, the problems of transferring such a system to other parts of the country will be substantial, particularly in metropolitan areas where there is a great deal of cross-boundary flow.

What counts as a referral?

Before data on numbers of referrals can be converted into referral rates to compare the behaviour of different doctors or practices, there needs to be agreement about what constitutes a referral. There are a number of areas where the definition of what constitutes a referral may be ambiguous.

The most clear-cut situation is where a GP writes to a hospital specialist asking for an appointment to be sent for an outpatient clinic. In the UK, patients generally have access to specialists only by referral from their GP. The few clinics to which patients can self-refer should not be included if the intention is to study GPs' referral patterns. If, on the other hand, the purpose is to examine the use of hospital services by a defined population, then self-referrals become very important, particularly for Accident and Emergency departments which sometimes provide substantial amounts of primary care, especially out of office hours and in large cities.

In the UK a specialist may arrange to follow-up a patient following an initial outpatient attendance. If a GP needs to expedite a pre-arranged follow-up appointment, this would not normally be regarded as a new referral. A further referral for the same problem following discharge from the specialist's clinic would normally be regarded as a new referral. These arrangements may be much less clear-cut in other countries (Chapter 3) in which the boundaries between doctors working in primary and secondary care may be more blurred.

A direct referral by a GP to a hospital outpatient department is under the control of the GP. Subsequently, the management of the patient is partly under the control of the specialist. The patient may be cross-referred to another specialist, or put on a waiting-list for inpatient admission. At present neither of these are conventionally included in discussion about GP referral rates. This again is appropriate if the purpose of data collection is to focus on the GP's behaviour, but the subsequent course of the patient will need to be included in any data collection system if the purpose is to measure the health care usage of the defined population made up by the GP's list of registered patients.

In any particular situation a decision needs to be made whether referrals to paramedical services and to specialists working in the community should be included. These are not included in either of the sets of referral data described above, though there are a number of services in the community to which GPs may have access and which may have a direct effect on referral patterns; for example, physiotherapy, community psychiatric nurses, and child health doctors. For many years there have been isolated examples of specialists carrying out clinics in practices, and this aspect of care may increase substantially as a result of the GP fundholding initiative. As the interaction between primary and secondary care evolves, new ways of sharing care between primary and secondary care may develop and it may be necesssary to review what the word referral actually means.

Counting diagnostic tests presents particular problems. Radiology is fairly straightforward as the patient usually attends the hospital for investigation, though it may be desirable to define whether diagnostic tests or patient attendances are being counted. Counting pathology tests is much more difficult. It is common to take a number of specimens when investigating a patient, and any one specimen may be used to order a number of different tests. The definition of 'a test' needs to be clear if figures from different practices are to be compared. One pragmatic approach would be to define the tests in terms of numbers of samples sent to the laboratory. Two tubes of blood from the same patient would therefore count as two tests even if they were sent to the same laboratory. There are probably fewer anomalies in this definition than in trying to count the number of analyses, as up to ten analyses may be carried out as part of one overall test request (for example, liver function tests, viral serology). An alternative would be to regard one set of specimens sent to any individual laboratory as 'one investigation'. Practices and HAs will need to decide the most effective method of recording the number of investigations carried out. From an administrative point of view, the simplest method may be to record the test when the results come back from the hospital.

Calculating referral rates — which denominator?

General practice in the UK is almost unique in that doctors are responsible for a defined population of patients registered with them. This means that a number of activities of the doctor can be defined in terms of the population served, and allows, for example, targets to be set for cervical cytology and immunization rates which would be impossible in most countries. The list size is therefore the natural denominator to use to measure referral rates.

However, the list size of an individual doctor in partnership may bear no relation to his workload. As an example, a new partner in an expanding practice may have only a few hundred patients registered with him personally while taking a full share of the workload. To use his list size as the denominator to calculate his referral rate would seriously underestimate his workload and produce an artificially high referral rate which would be meaningless. Likewise, a senior partner nearing retirement may have acquired a list of 3000 patients, but he may be gradually reducing his workload. Again his list size may bear little relation to the number of patients he sees. Indeed, trainees in general practice have no list of registered patients, so another denominator must be found to measure referral rates of trainees. List size, therefore, may be used as a denominator to measure referral rates of single-handed principals or of whole practices, but should not be used to measure referral rates of individual doctors within a group.

The average list size per partner has been suggested as a suitable denominator for calculating referral rates for individual doctors (Armstrong *et al.* 1988). Although this is preferable to using individual list sizes, it is still unsatisfactory because it assumes equal workload between partners, which is often not the case (Roland *et al.* 1989).

While referral rates based on a whole practice are valuable for comparing practices, they do not therefore provide sufficient information for doctors to look at their own individual performance. In order for a doctor to look at his own clinical behaviour the number of referrals he makes needs to be related in some way to his workload. The simplest way to do this is to use the number of consultations he undertakes as the denominator to calculate referral rates, which will then be expressed in terms of number of referrals per 100 consultations. Apart from problems of case mix discussed below, there is a potential difficulty in using consultations as the denominator, which relates to doctors' propensity to ask patients to return. Up to half of consultations in general practice may be initiated by the doctor himself for the follow-up of acute or chronic disease. Doctors probably vary greatly in the proportion of patients they ask to return, and the number of consultations carried out may therefore depend on the doctor's behaviour. For this reason the number of patients who consult has been proposed as a denominator as an alternative to the number of consultations, and many of the rates in the National Morbidity Surveys (RCGP/OPCS/DHSS 1986) are presented in this form. Although the number of patients consulting may have theoretical advantages over the number of consultations as a denominator for calculating referral rates the advantage is probably small (Roland *et al.* 1990) and the greatly increased complexity of data collection not generally worthwhile.

In summary, the most satisfactory way to calculate a referral rate for a practice is to divide the number of referrals by the practice list size, to give a rate conventionally expressed per 1000 patients on the list. For individual doctors, the most satisfactory rate is to divide the number of referrals by the number of consultations carried out by that doctor to give a rate, conventionally expressed per 100 consultations.

Calculating a referral rate: an example

Suppose Dr Jones and his partners refer 1650 patients to NHS hospitals during a year, of whom 144 are referred to the ENT clinic. Their list size was 10 050 in the middle of the year. Their overall NHS referral rate is 1650/10 050 × 1000 = 164.2 referrals/1000 patients/year. Their ENT referral rate is 144/10 050 × 1000 = 14.3 referrals/1000 patients/year.

Allowing for age differences between practices

Practices differ in age structure. If the differences are small then it is not worth worrying about them. However, one practice may provide care for a local college and have a large number of students, whereas an adjacent one may have as high proportion of retired and elderly patients. These differences complicate the interpretation of referral rates. As an example, if ophthalmology referrals are commoner in older patients, one would expect more referrals to this specialty from a practice with a high proportion of elderly patients. The ophthalmology referral rate for this practice could not therefore be validly compared with data from a practice with a smaller proportion of elderly patients. If such differences do exist then they can be allowed for by standardizing for age differences between practices. In order to do this it is necessary to know the age structure of practices one is trying to compare, and to know a standard set of age-related referral rates. A suitable set of rates derived from the Third National Morbidity Survey (RCGP/OPCS/DHSS 1986) is shown in Table 5.1.

If FHSAs are to feed back referral data to GPs, they would be wise to standardize for age. Since they already have access to practice structures in terms of age, the statistical calculations needed to control for age are simple. It is the experience of those who have been involved in feeding back referral information to GPs that one of the first things which doctors bring up is the age structure of their practice. Even if the effects of standardization are not very great, discussions are likely to proceed to a meaningful stage more quickly if age differences between practices have been allowed for in the calculation of rates. It is also possible to control for sex differences between practices, but there are likely to be few circumstances where this will be valuable.

Allowing for case mix

Doctors' referral patterns are likely to be affected substantially by the types of clinical problems which they see. When comparing the referral rates of whole practices, an assumption is made that, averaged out over a

Table 5.1 *Age-specific referral rates per 1000 registered patients. These rates are derived from Table 5 and Fiche Table 13A in the Third National Morbidity Survey (RCGP et al. 1986) Grouping into smaller age bands does not confer significant advantage over the table as shown.*

	All ages	0–14	15–64	65 and over
Orthopaedics	8.81	7.25	7.88	15.00
Psychiatry	5.35	1.50	5.89	8.47
Dermatology	7.85	5.63	8.27	9.20
ENT	8.34	12.03	6.29	11.88
Medicine	19.27	11.25	14.94	48.91
Rheumatology	8.43	2.18	9.98	10.64
Neurology	4.48	3.42	3.93	8.34
Gynaecology	9.48	0.43	13.97	3.04
Obstetrics	8.84	0.03	13.83	0.00
Surgery	15.26	8.21	14.92	26.70
Ophthalmology	6.42	5.74	4.54	15.41
GU	0.52	0.06	0.76	0.13
Urology	4.21	5.07	3.07	7.86
All specialties	117.54	74.3	119.6	175.62

sufficiently long period of time, the types of illness encountered by doctors in one practice will be broadly similar to those of their neighbours. The question of allowing for differences in the type of patient seen by different doctors becomes more relevant when one is trying to compare referral rates to individual specialties, and the problem is greatest when looking at the referral rates of individual doctors in a practice to one particular specialty. A referral rate based on the number of referrals to specialists divided by the number of consultations carried out by that GP will not reflect differences in the types of patients seen by different GPs. As an example, a female doctor may see an unusually high proportion of patients with gynaecological problems (Roland *et al.* 1990), or a doctor with particular clinical skills in other areas may selectively attract a particular type of patient either because patients learn of his expertise or because his partners refer patients to him (Reynolds *et al.* 1991).

Resolving this type of problem can only be done by collecting data within practices, and this may be the sort of data which doctors will be stimulated to collect in order to explore apparent differences in referral rates between partners. As an example, if one doctor in a practice has a particularly high rate of referral to rheumatology, he and his partners may wish to collect information on the number and type of rheumatological problems which they each see, and to discuss how they each manage common rheumatological problems.

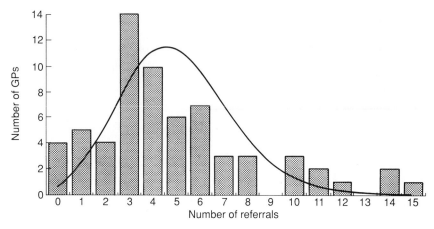

Fig. 5.1 Theoretical model based on Poisson distribution showing wide range of referral rates from GPs to outpatient departments predicted on the basis of chance alone. Histogram shows actual variation in numbers referred in a study by Dowie (1983): the solid line gives numbers predicted by the model (Moore and Roland 1989).

The problem of case mix may also be an issue when comparing the referral rates of different practices. We know that there are large differences in mortality, and therefore probably in morbidity, in different parts of the country. One would therefore expect differences in referral rates between different parts of the country as a result of clinical need. This area has yet to be explored in detail, and it is likely to be very complicated, partly because there may be other systematic differences between areas of high and low mortality, such as the type of doctor attracted to work in different areas, the availability of support services, and the expectations of patients, and these variables are likely to make it extremely difficult to isolate the role of doctors' behaviour when explaining overall variation in referral rates.

How much variation is due to chance?

Some of the variation in GPs' rates of referral to hospital may be due to random variation in the presentation of patients requiring referral. This is a particular problem when dealing with small numbers of referrals, to a single specialty over a limited period of time, for example, when the proportion of variation simply due to chance may be a substantial proportion of the observed variation in referral rates. Moore and Roland (1989) have described a mathematical model to calculate the amount of variation in rates or referral that is likely to be due to chance alone. Some examples are given below.

In Fig. 5.1 the histogram shows the range of numbers of referrals made

Table 5.2 *Variation in referral numbers likely to be due to chance*

	Average no of referrals	Expected range
Rheumatology, 1 GP, 6 months	5	0–10
Rheumatology, 5 GPs, 1 year	50	36–64
Gyneacology, 1 GP, 6 months	14	6–21
Gynaecology, 5 GPs, 1 year	137	114–160
General Surgery, 1 GP, 6 months	21	11–30
General Surgery, 5 GPs, 1 year	209	180–238
All specialties, 1 GP, 6 months	165	139–191
All specialties, 5 GPs, 1 year	1650	1577–1723

by 65 GPs to a general medical outpatient clinic over a 13-week period in a study by Dowie (1983). Four doctors referred no patients at all during this period, while one doctor referred 15. One the face of it this appears a very wide range of referral behaviour. However, the solid line on the graph shows the amount of variation which would have been expected to occur on the basis of chance alone in this situation. It can be seen that a substantial part of the variation observed by Dowie could have been due to chance owing to the relatively small number of referrals that were being studied.

Table 5.2 shows some examples of the variation in referral rates which might be expected to result from chance alone using Moore and Roland's model. Referral rates outside the range in the right-hand column have a less than 5 per cent chance of being so extreme simply as a result of chance. The figures in Table 5.2 are derived from average referral rates of East Anglian doctors to a number of different specialties, and assume an average list size of 2000 patients per doctor.

The figures in Table 5.2 emphasize the substantial amount of variation which may be due to chance when referrals relating to a single specialty or referral data collected over a short period of time are examined. The right hand column of Table 5.2 is analogous to a 95 per cent confidence limit for numbers of referrals. A table to allow confidence limits for referral rates to be looked up is shown in Appendix 1 of this chapter. In general, it is unwise to compare the referral rates of practices if the data are based on an average of less than 30 referrals per practice.

Example of calculation of confidence limits for referral rates

Dr Brown and her partners have 6000 patients, of whom they referred 28 to neurology over one year. Their neurology referral rate is 28/6000 × 1000 = 4.7 referrals per 1000 patients per year. In the whole HA area there are 1400 neurology referrals for a population of 500 000 patients, a rate of 2.8 referrals per 1000 patients per year. To calculate the confidence limits for a practice of Dr Brown's size, look down the left-hand vertical axis of Appendix 1 until you come to 3 (nearest to 2.8), and across until you come to a list size of 6000, to give a figure of 2. The confidence limit for neurology referrals for a practice of Dr Brown's size is therefore 2.8 ± 2, i.e. 0.8–4.8. Dr Brown's practice comes within this range, so they should not be regarded as significantly high referrers even though their neurology referral rate is well above the average for the HA area.

One way to avoid this problem of wide confidence intervals due to small numbers of referrals is to group specialties together. On the whole, a year's data will only allow referral rates to be calculated reliably for the largest specialties. For smaller specialties, there are often natural groupings which should be used when calculating referral rates. As examples, under general medicine include gastroenterology, thoracic medicine, endocrinology, cardiology, infectious diseases, and renal medicine; under general surgery include urology; under rheumatology include physical medicine and rehabilitation; under psychiatry include mental handicap and psychotherapy.

In Appendix 2 of this chapter a further statistical method for handling referral rates is described. This method partitions the overall variation in referral rates across a number of specialties into random and systematic components. The random component is that part of the variation which is likely to be due to chance. The systematic component is that part which is likely to be due to some other factor; for example, a difference in the morbidity of patients or a difference in doctors' referral behaviour. The particular value of the method described in Appendix 2 is that it allows the systematic variation in referral rates to be compared across a range of specialties with different average referral rates. In relation to medical audit, a HA might well wish to focus attention on those specialties in which referral rates seemed particularily variable. Appendix 2 shows how this may be done, allowing for the variation which is due to chance.

When is variation in referral rates important?

In the previous section the importance of random variation in referral rates based on small numbers of referrals has been discussed. However, for large numbers of referrals — for example, a whole practice's referrals over one year — the statistical variation due to chance may be quite small. Therefore, in addition to calculating statistical significance it is important to decide whether variation in referral rates is practically significant. There is no point in telling the doctors in a practice that they are significantly high referrers if, from a practical point of view, their referral rates are not all that different from those of their peers. This is particularly important if it has not been possible to take into account some of the factors which may substantially affect the figures; for example, private referrals. The amount of variation which is practically significant is a matter of judgement, but it would probably be unwise to draw the attention of practices to their referral rates unless those rates lay outside at least a twofold range around the average value for doctors in that HA area.

Conclusion

The development of methods of collecting routine data about hospital referrals will have benefits, both in terms of being able to analyse geographical patterns of hospital referral, and by allowing the calculation of referral rates for individual practices. The issues described in this chapter demonstrate that considerable care needs to be taken in the calculation and interpretation of referral rates, particularily as the quality of data currently being collected in the National Health Service is very variable. Nevertheless routine collection of data about hospital referrals is a necessary first step if doctors are to be in a position constructively to examine their referral patterns.

This chapter has concentrated on methods of analysing referral data without reference to what referral rates actually mean. It is important to understand that there is at present no clear relationship between a doctor's rate of referral to hospital and the quality of care that he provides for his patients. However, referral rates may be used as a tool to encourage doctors to look critically at the care they provide both for patients referred to hospital and for those not referred, and these issues are discussed further in Chapters 10 and 11.

Appendix 1

The figures give the range of variation one would expect to occur by chance for each average rate shown in the left hand column. As an example, if the average referral rate for a specialty is 25/1000 patients per year across a whole HA area, the 95 per cent confidence interval for a practice of 2000 would be 7 patients per 1000 per year. The practice could therefore be expected to refer at a rate between 18 and 32 per 1000 per year (25 +/- 7). Since there are 2000 patients on the list, the number of referrals could range from 36–64 patients entirely by chance.

FHSA rate/1000 pts/year	List size									
	250	500	1000	2000	4000	6000	8000	10 000	12 000	16 000
1	4	3	2	2	1	1	1	1	1	1
3	6	4	3	3	2	2	1	1	1	1
5	9	5	4	3	3	2	2	1	1	1
10	14	9	7	5	3	3	2	2	2	2
15	17	12	8	6	4	3	3	3	3	2
20	19	14	9	6	4	4	3	3	3	2
25	21	16	10	7	5	4	4	3	3	2
30	23	17	11	8	5	4	4	3	3	3
40	26	19	12	9	6	5	4	4	4	3
50	29	21	14	10	7	6	5	4	4	3
60	31	23	15	11	8	7	5	5	4	4
70	33	25	16	12	8	7	6	5	5	4
80	37	26	18	13	9	7	6	6	5	4
90	39	27	19	13	9	8	7	6	5	5
100	41	29	20	14	10	8	7	6	6	5
120	44	30	21	15	11	9	8	7	6	5
140	48	33	23	17	12	10	8	7	7	6
160	50	37	25	18	13	10	9	8	7	6
180	53	39	26	19	13	11	9	8	8	7
200	56	41	28	20	14	11	10	9	8	7
220	58	43	29	21	15	12	10	9	8	7
240	61	44	30	22	15	12	11	10	9	8
270	65	47	32	23	16	13	11	10	9	8
300	68	49	34	24	17	14	12	11	10	9
400	80	56	41	28	20	17	14	12	11	10
500	88	62	44	30	22	18	15	13	12	12
600	104	68	49	34	24	20	17	15	14	13
800	112	80	56	41	28	24	20	18	17	14
1000	124	88	62	44	30	26	22	20	18	15

Appendix 2

If there were no systematic differences between doctors in referral rates, there would still be random variation. The method described here separates the overall variation in rates into random variation and systematic variation between doctors. The systematic variation, including that due to variation in decisions by doctors, can be found by subtracting the random variation from the overall variation.

This calculation can be carried out separately for each specialty to determine which are subject to greatest non-random variation.

For practice j let the actual (observed) number of referrals = $O_{(j)}$

Let the expected number of referrals (if the practice referred at the same rate as the FHSA average = $E_{(j)}$

where $E_{(j)}$ = the number of patients in practice j × referral rate/1000 for the whole FHSA.

If there are k practices, then

$$\text{random variation} = \frac{1}{k} \sum_{j=1}^{k} \frac{1}{E_j}$$

$$\text{and total variation} = \frac{1}{k} \sum_{j=1}^{k} \left(\frac{O_j - E_j}{E_j} \right)^2 .$$

Systematic variation = total variation − random variation.

This method of calculating the systematic component of variation between practices is independent of the absolute number of referrals. The relative variation between a number of specialties can therefore be directly compared. Doctors or practices whose expected number of referrals is less than 5 should be omitted from the calculations.

Two statistical tests may be used to assess the significance of the variation. The ratio of the systematic component of variation within a specialty to the random component can be compared on the F distribution on $k-1$, $k-1$ degrees of freedom, where k is the number of practices. This will indicate whether the systematic variation between doctors' referral rates to that specialty is greater than would be expected by chance. Thus

systematic variation/random variation is distributed as $F_{k-1, k-1}$.

The F test can also be used to compare the systematic components of variation for two specialities, to indicate whether variability in referral rates is greater in one speciality than in another. Thus

systematic variation for specialty j/systematic variation for specialty i
is distributed as $F_{k-1, m-1}$ where k and m are the numbers of practices
used to calculate the variation for specialties j and i respectively.

This method was described by McPherson *et al.* (1982). Its application to referral data is described by Roland *et al.* (1990).

References

Armstrong, D., Britten, N., and Grace, J. (1988). Measuring general practitioners' referrals: patient workload and list size. *Journal of the Royal College of General Practitioners* **38**, 494–7.

Coulter, A., Noone, A., and Goldacre, M. (1989). General practitioners' referrals to specialist outpatient clinics. II: Location of specialist outpatient clinics to which general practitioners refer patients. *British Medical Journal* **299**, 306–8.

Coulter, A., Roland, M.O., and Wilkin, D. (1991). *GP referrals to hospital: a guide for Family Health Services Authorities.* Centre for Primary Care Research, Manchester.

Department of Health and Social Security (1987). *Promoting better health.* HMSO, London.

Dowie, R. (1983). *General practitioners and consultants — a study of outpatient referrals.* King Edward's Hospital Fund for London, London.

McPherson, K., Wennberg, J.E., Hovind, O.B., and Clifford, P. (1982). Small area variations in the use of common surgical procedures: an international comparison of New England, England and Norway. *New England Journal of Medicine* **307**, 1310–14.

Moore, A.T. and Roland, M.O. (1989). How much variation in referral rates among general practitioners is due to chance? *British Medical Journal* **298**, 500–2.

Reynolds, D., Chitnis, J.G., and Roland, M.O. (1991). General practitioner referrals: do good doctors refer more patients to hospital? *British Medical Journal* **302**, 1250–2.

Roland, M.O., Middleton, J., Goss, B., and Moore, A.T. (1989). Should performance indicators in general practice relate to whole practices or to individual doctors. *Journal of the Royal College of General Practitioners* **39**, 461–2.

Roland, M.O., Bartholomew, J., Morrell, D.C., McDermott, A., and Paul, E. (1990). Understanding hospital referral rates: a user's guide. *British Medical Journal* **301**, 98–102.

Royal College of General Practitioners Office of Population Censuses and Surveys, Department of Health and Social Security (1986). *Morbidity statistics from general practice 1981–2: third national study.* HMSO, London.

6 Patterns of referral: explaining variation

David Wilkin

Introduction

One of the most consistent findings in general practice research is the existence of wide variations in all aspects of care. Patients looked after by different GPs experience different patterns of consultations, prescribing, use of investigations, referral to specialists, and so on. In our own studies of 200 GPs in greater Manchester we reported that consultation rates ranged from less than two per patient per year to more than five, prescribing rates from less than 50 per 100 consultations to more than 90, investigation rates from less than one per 100 consultations to more than 15, referral rates from less than three per 100 consultations to more than 17 (Wilkin *et al.* 1987). Even after making allowance for sampling error it is quite clear that wide variations do exist between GPs. The fact that similar variations exist in hospital practice, and indeed in the practice of other professionals, should not deter us from further investigation of the possible causes and consequences of differences in the care provided by GPs. We need to know whether such wide variations matter in terms of outcomes for patients and what factors might account for variation.

Perhaps not surprisingly, attention to variations in GP care has focused on those aspects which have the greatest cost implications; prescribing, use of investigations, and referral to hospital. Politicians and health service managers have understandably been concerned to know whether economies could be achieved through more rational use of drugs, hospital services, and laboratory and X-ray facilities. They have looked at the wide variations between GPs and asked whether these could be justified in terms of the needs of patients. If not, they argued, pressure should be brought to bear on high users to reduce their use and thus achieve substantial savings. This approach has provided the basis for reviews of GP prescribing behaviour including the current PACT system, which provides doctors with detailed information on their own prescribing as compared with that of their colleagues. During the past five years they have increasingly turned their attention to patterns of GP referral to specialists.

In 1985 the Chief Medical Officer of the Department of Health Sir Donald Acheson (1985) expressed his concern at the wide variation in GP referral rates and his frustration that 'a phenomenon so gross can continue to defy analysis'. He highlighted both variations between GPs and between different parts of the country. The theme has been pursued in subsequent government white papers (Secretaries of State for Social Services, Wales, Northern Ireland and Scotland 1987, 1989) and most recently in the report by the National Audit Office (1991) on NHS out-patient services. This latter report is somewhat more cautious than earlier documents in pointing out that variations in referral rates raise questions concerning the quality of care and whether resources are being used efficiently and effectively. The authors accept that until more information is available it would be unwise to draw conclusions.

The purpose of this chapter is to summarize and review what we know to date about patterns of GP referral and the extent to which we are able to explain variations between doctors. Inevitably this exercise will identify large gaps in our knowledge and understanding, so that the concluding dis-cussion will focus on what needs to be done to improve the position. This discussion will be placed in the context of the changes currently being im-plemented in the NHS, although most of the points made are applicable regardless of the particular financial and managerial arrangements.

Describing patterns of referral

Referral rates

Most of the research which contributes to our knowledge of patterns of referral has focused on global rates, often to the exclusion of other considerations. A range of both large and small studies enable us to construct a reasonable picture of overall rates of referral. The average rate of referral to hospital-based specialists is between four and six per 100 consultations or between 10 and 12 per 100 registered patients per year, although Table 6.1 shows considerable differences between studies in their estimates of the overall rate. The largest study available to date, the third National morbidity study (RCGP/OPCS 1986), reported a rate of 11.8 referrals per 100 population and 3.5 per 100 consultations. These rates are low in comparison to those reported in other studies. They are also very low in comparison to many other countries, where far more medical care is provided by specialists (Chapter 3). In the NHS the gatekeeper system works very effectively, so that the vast majority of illness episodes presenting to the GP are dealt with at that level.

There is also general agreement among studies that there is wide vari-ation between GPs in their referral rates. There is, however, less agree-ment concerning the extent of this variation. At one extreme the Chief Medical Officer has expressed concern over an apparent twentyfive-fold variation in GP referral rates (Acheson 1985), but Moore and Roland (1989) have pointed out that much of the observed variation may be accounted for by chance, since all of the studies to date have been based

Table 6.1 *Comparison of referral rates from selected studies*

Author and reference	Dates of data collection	Number of practices/ doctors	Type(s) of referrals	Number of consultations	Number of referrals	Referral rate Mean	Range	Comments
Barber (1971)	1970	1 GP	Outpatient inc referrals to opticians and dentists	6008	219	3.6 per 100 consultations		Methods inadequately described
Fry (1972)	1972	2 GPs	Referral to hospital	18 915[a]	360[a]	4.0 per 100 patients on list		[a]Calculated from quoted figures
Crombie (1984)	1971/2	39 practices	Hospital			3.3 per 100 consultations (median)	1.9–6.4	Data derived from second national morbidity study
Marsh and McNay (1974)	1972	1 GP	Outpatients and inpatients	7272[b]	376[b]	5.2 per 100 consultations[b]; 12.0 per 100 patients on list per year[b]		[b]Calculated from quoted figures
Fraser (1974)	1970	18 GPs	All hospital referrals	33 000 (approx)	1068	3.2 per 100 consultations		No comparison of doctors provided
JR CGP (1978)	1977	100 GPs	Outpatient, domiciliary, and admissions	64 986	2755	3.4 per 100 consultations (outpatient); 4.2 per 100 consultations (total)	1.7–9.8	

Cummins (1981)	1974–1978	5 GPs	Outpatient	65 538	3545	5.4 per 100 consultations; 13.2 per 100 patients on list per year	4.3–6.7	
Gillam (1985)	1982	18 GPs	Outpatient and domiciliary visits	27 847	898	3.1 per 100 consultations	1.8–5.6	
Wilkin and Smith (1987a)	1981/2	201 GPs	All referrals to consultants	89 030	5467	6.1 per 100 consultations	1.0–24.0	
RCGP and OPCS (1986)	1981/2	48 practices 143 GPs	All referrals	1 045 341	36 162	11.8 per 100 patients per year 3.5 per 100 consultations	Not provided	Third national morbidity study
			Outpatient			7.9 per 100 patients per year 2.3 per 100 consultations	Not provided	
Jones (1987)	1985	Not reported	Outpatient	Not collected	48 000	20 per 100 population per year	7.3–41.5 (practices)	Based on survey of outpatient clinics Includes non-GP referrals

Table 6.1 (*continued*)

Author and reference	Dates of data collection	Number of practices/ doctors	Type(s) of referrals	Number of consultations	Number of referrals	Referral rate Mean	Range	Comments
Armstrong and Griffin (1987) Armstrong, Britten, and Grace (1988)	1982	122 GPs	Outpatient	17 445	967	5.5 per 100 consultations	Not provided	Discrepancies between rates reported in two papers
Noone et al. (1989)	1983	8 practices 17 practices	Outpatient Outpatient	Not collected	1146 3517	10.2 10.1	8.4–18.1 6.9–16.4	Rates are standardized for age and sex
	1984	8 practices 17 practices	Outpatient Outpatient		1382 3723	11.4 10.4 per 100 patients per year	6.7–15.9 5.1–15.1	
Madeley et al. (1990)	1987	34 practices	Outpatient	Not collected	3534	9.6 per 100 patients per year	2.8–17.6	Based on outpatient records at one hospital
Reynolds et al. (1991)	1989	6 GPs	Outpatient	21 784 surgery consultations	612	2.8 per 100 consultations	1.6–3.9	

on relatively small samples (Chapter 5). Those studies summarized in Table 6.1 which report ranges of referral rates for individual GPs or practices all indicate substantial variation in gross rates, however these are calculated. Studies based on larger numbers of referrals using longer recording periods tend to show somewhat less variation. Also, calculating rates for practices rather than individual GPs has the effect of reducing the extent of variation observed since differences between doctors within the same practice are ironed out. Moore and Roland (1989) point out that the substantial element of random variation has the effect of concealing real differences, making interpretation and explanation of causes more difficult. It is to be hoped that continuing debate about the extent of variation in rates of referral will be resolved as the results of much larger-scale studies become available.

On the basis of the evidence to date it seems safe to assume that the real variation in GP referral rates is at least threefold or fourfold. Average referral rates for the upper and lower quintiles in our study of 201 GPs were 11.8 and 2.9 per hundred consultations respectively (Wilkin and Smith 1987a). Crombie and Fleming (1988) found a fourfold variation between practices in the National Morbidity Studies and Noone *et al.* (1989) reported a threefold variation among 25 practices in the Oxford region. Patients registered with high-referring practices are thus three times more likely to see a specialist than those registered with low referrers.

Distribution between specialties

Variations between GPs in gross referral rates have tended to attract most attention in the published literature, often to the exclusion of other issues. In particular there is relatively little evidence concerning the distribution of referrals between the different specialties and the extent to which this varies. This is to some extent because the numbers required to calculate specialty-specific referral rates are beyond the scope of individual research projects. However, as more sophisticated information systems become available it will be important to look at the extent to which GPs vary in their use of different specialties.

Table 6.2 shows the broad distribution of referrals between selected specialties in six health districts in greater Manchester. In this study 372 GPs each recorded information on 30 consecutive referrals to specialists. The distribution of referrals between specialties varied from one district to another. Thus, for example, only 8 per cent of referrals in District D were to specialists in general medicine, compared with 14 per cent in District B. Only 2 per cent of referrals in District F were to a psychiatrist, compared with 6 per cent in District B. Combining surgical specialties (general surgery, gynaecology, ENT, and orthopaedics) 53 per cent of

Table 6.2 *Distribution of referrals between selected specialties for six districts (percentages)*

District	A	B	C	D	E	F	Total
Number of referrals (100 per cent)	1324	1427	1955	2270	1670	1641	10 287
Specialty:							
General surgery	16	16	17	20	20	18	18
General medicine	11	14	10	8	10	11	10
Gynaecology	11	10	10	10	10	10	10
Ear, nose, and throat surgery	10	8	9	9	11	10	9
Orthopaedics	8	7	8	14	12	12	10
Ophthalmology	5	4	4	6	6	7	5
Dermatology	5	4	5	7	5	5	5
Paediatrics	5	4	5	3	5	4	4
Geriatric medicine	3	4	3	2	1	2	2
Psychiatry	4	6	4	3	3	2	4

referrals in Districts D and E were to surgeons, compared with only 41 per cent in District B and 44 per cent in District C. There are no grounds for supposing that patients' needs for surgical intervention differed systematically between districts. Unfortunately, the number of referrals per GP in this study is insufficient to calculate specialty-specific rates for individual doctors and therefore to look at patterns of variation. Although we lack clear evidence of the extent of variation between GPs in their use of different specialties, there is some evidence that gross referral rates are reflected in the pattern of referrals between specialties, so that high referrers tend to refer more patients to all specialties, rather than concentrating their referrals in particular specialties (Wilkin and Smith 1986).

Other aspects of referral

Other aspects of the referral decision might also be expected to show variations between doctors. Thus decisions have to be made about the mode of referral (inpatient, outpatient, domiciliary visit) and about the urgency attached to it. Given the wide variations observed in referral rates we might expect these aspects of the referral decision to be equally variable. As for specialty-specific rates, we do not yet have adequate data on the extent of variation between GPs, but there are clearly differences between districts.

Table 6.3 shows the overall pattern for six health districts for selected specialties. GPs in District F were more likely to seek admission to hospital than their colleagues in Districts A and E, but those in Districts A and B were more likely to refer through accident and emergency departments.

Table 6.3 *Mode of referral and urgency for six districts (percentages)*

District	A	B	C	D	E	F	Total
Number of referrals (100 per cent)	1324	1427	1955	2270	1670	1641	10 287
Mode of referral:							
Out patient	92	89	91	92	92	88	91
In-patient (Admission)	3	5	5	6	4	8	5
Accident & Emergency	4	4	2	1	3	2	2
Domiciliary Visits	1	2	2	1	1	2	1
Urgency:							
Routine	78	72	78	78	80	69	76
Urgent	15	19	15	16	13	21	16
Immediate	7	9	7	6	7	10	8

Doctors in districts B and F were more likely to label their referrals 'urgent' or requiring 'immediate attention'. Thus there is some evidence from these figures of considerable variations in other aspects of referral. Although attention has focused largely on rates of referral, it is important to bear in mind that there are other important ways in which the referral patterns of GPs will differ.

Explaining variations

Faced with substantial variations in GP referral rates, two key questions immediately arise. Why should these variations exist and what consequences do they have for patients and for the health service? Most attention to date has been devoted to the first of these. Factors which have been advanced as possible explanations of variations can be divided into three broad categories; patient variables, provider variables, and health care system variables.

Patient variables

The most obvious explanation for differences in rates of referral is that they simply reflect differences in need. Clearly, consultations with some categories of patients (for example, elderly people, women of child-bearing age, and those with certain chronic conditions) generate relatively large numbers of referrals to specialists. It might therefore be expected that the patients of high-referring GPs would include a disproportionate representation of such groups.

In our study we compared the age and sex of patients consulting high- and low-referring doctors and found them to be very similar (Wilkin and

Smith 1987*a*). Information on social class is more difficult to collect and interpret. Crombie (1984) showed a gradient in referral rates for males per 100 population, with the lowest in social class I and the highest in social class V. In contrast, Morrell *et al.* (1971) reported that rates per 100 population rose from class V to class I. This was confirmed by Cummins *et al.* (1981) and in our own study (Wilkin and Smith 1987*a*). However, Cummins reported that the class gradient was reversed if allowance was made for the higher consultation rates of lower social classes.

The most recent evidence from the socio-economic analyses of the third National Morbidity Study (McCormick and Rosenbaum 1991) shows no clear pattern. In 1981/2 men in social class I and II were slightly less likely to be referred than those in classes IV and V, but those in III non-manual and III manual had the highest rate of referral. Among women, the highest rate was found among those in social classes IV an V and the lowest in class III non-manual. However, in all cases the differences between classes in standardized referral ratios were small. It is worth noting that this latest volume of tables from the third National Morbidity Study includes much detailed information on the relationships between referral rates, social class, and other socio-economic variables (for example, marital status, housing tenure, employment) which warrants further analysis. To date, however, the evidence on social class gradients in referral rates remains unclear. Not surprisingly, therefore, differences in the social class composition of patient populations do not appear to account for variations in individual GP referral rates.

Perhaps the sharpest variations in referral rates occur between different diagnostic groups. Thus the third National Morbidity Study showed that referrals for outpatient appointments ranged from 2.4 per cent of patients consulting for diseases of the respiratory system to 33 per cent of patients consulting for neoplasms (RCGP/OPCS 1986). In the light of this observation it seems possible that at least part of the variation between GPs might be accounted for by differences in the types of problems seen, since GPs in partnerships may be specializing in certain aspects of clinical work. However, our analyses of the case mix of patients seen by high and low referrers showed no differences in the range or distribution of problems seen (Wilkin and Smith 1986).

We also looked at whether high rates might reflect particular areas of expertise or lack of expertise. If this were so, it may be that high referrers lack expertise in certain areas of clinical work (or have a particular interest in/awareness of certain types of conditions) which generate large numbers of referrals. In the event we showed that high and low referrers behaved similarly across all conditions. Other researchers have confirmed this finding. Morrell *et al.* (1971) produced referral rates adjusted separately for age, sex, and social class and showed that these factors reduced only marginally the differences between doctors. Cummins *et al.* (1981)

adjusted simultaneously for age, sex, and social class with the same effect and also examined differences between doctors for six specific disorders.

The evidence to date fails to provide any substantial support for the hypothesis that differences between GPs in their referral rates reflect differences in the needs or characteristics of their patients. It seems that GPs at either end of the referral spectrum are seeing essentially the same types of patients with the same range of problems.

Provider variables

If variations in referral rates do not reflect differences in the patients seen or their needs for medical care, do they reflect systematic differences in the characteristics of the doctors and/or their practices? A host of possible explanatory variables has been suggested in the literature at various times (Wilkin and Smith 1987*b*). Among the most commonly advanced doctor characteristics are knowledge and experience. It has been suggested that younger, less experienced doctors are more likely to refer, but although Evans and McBride (1968) suggested that older doctors made less use of hospital services than their younger colleagues other studies have not supported this view. Wright's (1968) study of 68 doctors and Forsyth and Logan's (1968) study of 369 GPs showed no relationship between age and referral rate. Our own study indicated that high referrers included a greater proportion of experienced doctors than low referrers, but the differences were small (Wilkin and Smith 1987*a*). Contrary to popular belief, there was no evidence that more experienced doctors made less use of hospital services.

There are no simple indicators which would allow one to test the hypothesis that referral rates reflect differences in knowledge. However, various authors have suggested that background, training, and specialist interests might account for at least some of the variation. The only available evidence suggests no clear relationship. Forsyth and Logan (1968) showed that GPs who held clinical assistantships in hospitals had rates of referral which were much the same as their colleagues, and that degrees and diplomas held bore no relationship to referral behaviour. High and low referrers in our study included almost identical proportions who were members of the Royal College of General Practitioners and who held hospital appointments (Wilkin and Smith 1987*a*). However, a more recent study conducted in one group practice of five partners showed that doctors with particular experience in otorhinolarynology and opthalmology had higher rates of referral to these specialties, even after allowing for case mix (Reynolds *et al.* 1991).

It has been suggested that the structural features of practices, such as number of partners, ancillary staff, or number of patients, might be expected to have a bearing on referral rates. Although Forsyth and Logan's (1968) early study suggested that single-handed doctors had lower referral rates than those in partnerships, our data provides no support for this (Wilkin and Smith 1987*a*). Wright (1968) showed that GPs with small patient lists made more use of hospital outpatient departments, but Forsyth and Logan (1968) found no relationship between referral rates and list size, and this was supported by Scott and Gilmore (1966). In contrast Starey (1961) reported that rates were higher for lists over 3000 than for lists below 2000. In our study other practice characteristics such as the amount of ancillary help in the practice, the use of appointment systems, or the type of practice premises were all unrelated to referral rates (Wilkin and Smith 1987*a*).

The evidence concerning the ability of provider characteristics to explain variations in referral rates is inconclusive. However, it seems highly unlikely that, even with larger data sets, the sorts of variables considered to date will account for more than a tiny fraction of the variance between GPs. This should not be taken to imply that provider characteristics are unimportant, merely that those which are most easily measurable are unlikely to explain the differences. More recent research on the issue has begun to look at psychological variables which might be involved (Wilkin and Dornan 1990). Attitudes to risk and tolerance of uncertainty are being explored in a number of studies, and these seem to hold out a much better prospect of success than the relatively crude quantitative variables which have been looked at to date.

Health care system variables

Apart from patient and provider characteristics, a number of other factors have been suggested as possible contributors to variations in referral rates. These are mainly concerned with the availability and accessibility of hospital services. There are substantial regional variations in outpatient attendances which do not seem to be explicable in terms of differences in needs. Rather, they seem to reflect differences in the supply of outpatient clinics. However, they do not account for differences between GPs since there is much more variation within regions than between regions.

At a more local level there is also little evidence that GP referral rates are markedly influenced by the availability and accessibility of hospital services. Noone *et al.* (1989) were able to compare referral rates before and after the opening of a district general hospital in the new town of Milton Keynes, and to compare rates in the Milton Keynes area with rates of practices located elsewhere in the Oxford region. Although there was a small increase in rates following the opening of the hospital, the authors noted that variations between practices were far greater than variations between areas. Within a large urban area our own research showed that proximity to hospitals did not account for any of the variation between GPs in their referral rates (Wilkin and Smith 1986). At a national level Roland and Morris (1988) showed that the number of outpatients seen in medicine, thoracic medicine, psychiatry, and dermatology was strongly associated with the provision of consultants in these specialties.

There is some evidence that there are systematic differences in referral rates between GPs in rural and urban areas which may reflect differences in the accessibility of hospitals. In the third National Morbidity Study referrals in urban areas constituted 14 per cent of person years at risk compared with 9 per cent in rural areas (McCormick and Rosenbaum 1991). Similarly, Madeley *et al.* (1990) reported referral rates of 11 per 100 patients per year for urban practices compared with 8 for rural practices. However, it should be remembered that differences between GPs within areas far outweigh these difference between areas.

There are a number of other health system variables which might be expected to affect patterns of referral; for example, waiting times for appointment, range of services available, access to specific diagnostic or therapeutic services, organizational features of the service offered by specialists, and so on. However, although these might account for regional and area variations in referral rates or patterns of referral, they do not account for the variations between GPs, since these remain large within areas where all of the above conditions are the same for local GPs and their patients.

Consequences of variation

In the light of how much has been written on the subject of GP variation in referral rates, it is somewhat surprising that we know very little about the consequences of variation. To what extent do observations of differences in referral rates tell us anything about the effectiveness and efficiency of our health care? Are some patients failing to receive specialist treatment from which they would benefit whilst others are being treated unnecessarily, with possible adverse consequences in terms of iatrogenic disease? Are we wasting scarce hospital resources in treating patients whose problems could be dealt with at least as well in general practice?

Information on referral rates or patterns of referral on its own is not sufficient to answer these questions. We do not know what is a desirable referral rate, whether high-referring doctors refer more patients unnecessarily than those with low rates, or whether low-referring doctors are failing to refer patients who would benefit from specialist treatment. In order to be able to address these issues it is essential to know much more about the relationship between rates of referral and the appropriateness of referrals (Wilkin *et al.* 1989). This requires research on outcomes both for those patients who are referred to hospital and those who remain under the care of their GP. To date, research in this area has been limited to looking at intermediate outcomes, such as how worthwhile the GP felt the referral to have been (Brown 1979; Gillam 1985), what investigations or treatments were ordered by the hospital (Emmanuel and Walter 1989), or what investigations/treatment could have been initiated by the GP rather than the hospital (Ross *et al.* 1983). Current research in the UK is beginning to grapple with the problems of assessing health outcomes for patients referred and those not referred, but it will be some years before we have even limited information about the relationship between referral rates and patient outcomes.

Aside from the issue of patient outcomes, the main focus of interest in terms of the consequences of GP variations in referral rates has been their impact on efficiency. Since specialist hospital-based health care is far more costly than primary care, there is considerable incentive to ensure that patients are not referred unnecessarily. Crombie and Fleming (1988) have estimated the financial implications of GP variability in referral rates. They calculated that in 1981 £287 000 was spent on hospital services for the average practice population. They estimated that the hospital costs generated by a GP at the 80th centile of the referral rate distribution would be £365 000 per year, compared with £195 000 for a GP at the 20th centile of the distribution. However, it should be remembered that these calculations are based on crude average costs for all outpatient attendances. We do not currently have any information concerning differences in the costs per patient referred by GPs with widely differing referral rates.

Some politicians and health service managers have made the mistaken assumption that reducing variations in referral rates would reduce costs and increase efficiency. Whilst from the point of view of costs it is tempting to concentrate on reducing the rates of high-referring doctors, reducing variation also implies an increase in the number referred by those at the other end of the spectrum. If the number of referrals 'saved' at one end of the spectrum approximates the new referrals at the other, then the effect on costs is negligible, assuming that each referral costs the same. In practice this assumption may be dangerous. It is at least plausible that the referrals 'saved' will be of a relatively low cost, whereas the new referrals may well consist of patients who require substantial expenditure on investigation and treatment. If this is so the net effect of reducing variation could be an increase in the costs of secondary care. Lastly, if we have little information about cost, we have even less about efficiency. Because we know nothing about the appropriateness of referrals or their outcomes for patients, we do not know whether wide variations in patterns of referral are a sign of inefficiency or whether reducing this variation will increase efficiency.

Conclusions

Despite the considerable volume of published research on the subject of variations in patterns of referral and the obvious concerns of managers and politicians over this issue, there are relatively few clear conclusions which can be drawn to date. We know that there are wide variations in the rates at which GPs refer patients to specialists, although these are unlikely to be as wide as has sometimes been claimed. The results of large-scale studies should provide precise figures in the near future, but it seems likely that these will show variation in overall rates of the order of threefold or fourfold. More importantly, research based on computerized information systems should provide much more information on specialty-specific rates and other aspects of the pattern of referrals, such as the mode of referral, urgency, and subsequent investigation and treatment.

The lack of precision in measuring the true extent of variation and the inability of many studies to distinguish between random variation and systematic differences has contributed to our inability to explain variations. Most of the research findings to date are negative in the sense of excluding a variety of factors which might have been expected to contribute to variation. Thus patient characteristics, practice structure, and doctor characteristics have all failed to explain more than a tiny fraction of the variation. Whether more accurate measurement of rates based on larger numbers will produce different answers remains to be seen, but seems doubtful. The selection of independent variables has largely been based on what was readily available or easily collected, rather than on what might be considered theoretically most important. If we are to make progress in identifying those factors which influence GPs' propensity to refer to specialists, and therefore their referral rates, it will be essential to start from an appreciation of the referral decision. What factors are involved in the decision and how might these affect referral thresholds? The most promising research in this field is beginning to look at psychological and social variables, often using qualitative methods to explore the complexities of the decision-making process.

Perhaps the most important developments from the point of view of both research and management lie in the field of information systems. It seems inconceivable in an age of information technology that even basic information about the numbers of patients referred to hospital should have to be collected manually. Nevertheless, this is still the situation in some areas. HAs and hospitals are now developing outpatient information systems, but even these will not provide record linkage which would permit patients to be followed through from primary care to hospital outpatient department to inpatient care. Only through the provision of truly linked information systems will it be possible to monitor referral patterns accurately and to begin to examine their impact on costs, patterns of treatment, and patient outcomes.

This chapter has focused on the issue of GP variation in patterns of referral, more specifically referral rates, the extent to which this can be explained and its possible consequences. This emphasis reflects both concerns within the British NHS and the information currently available.

It should, however, be noted that this is only one facet of the interface between primary and secondary care, and that concentrating on differences between GPs in their crude rates of referral tells us nothing about the care actually provided at primary or secondary levels, its appropriateness, or the health outcomes for patients.

References

Acheson, D. (1985). Variation in GP referral rates still unexplained. *General Practitioner* Nov 8th.

Armstrong, D. and Griffin, G.A. (1987). Patterns of work in general practice in the Bromley health district. *Journal of the Royal College of General Practitioners* **37**, 264–6.

Armstrong, D., Britten, N., and Grace, J. (1988). Measuring general practitioner referrals: patient, workload and list size effects. *Journal of the Royal College of General Practitioners* **38**, 494–7.

Barber, J.H. (1971). Computer assisted recording in general practice. *Journal of the Royal College of General Practitioners* **21**, 726–36.

Brown, J.M. (1979). Why not audit hospital referrals? *Journal of the Royal College of General Practitioners* **29**, 743.

Crombie, D.L. (1984). Social class and health status inequality or difference. *Royal College of General Practitioners Occasional Paper No. 25*. Royal College of General Practitioners, Exeter.

Crombie, D.L. and Fleming, D.M. (1988). General practitioner referrals to hospital: the financial implications of variability. *Health Trends* **20**, 53–6.

Cummins, R.O., Jarman, B., and White, P.M. (1981). Do general practitioners have different 'referral thresholds'? *British Medical Journal* **282**, 1037–9.

Emmanuel, J. and Walter, N. (1989). Referrals from general practice to hospital outpatient departments: a strategy for improvement. *British Medical Journal* **299**, 722–4.

Evans, E.O. and McBride, K. (1968). Hospital usage by a group practice. *Journal of the Royal College of General Practitioners* **16**, 294–306.

Forsyth, G. and Logan, R.F.L. (1968). *Gateway or dividing line? A study of hospital outpatients in the 1960s*. Oxford University Press, Oxford.

Fraser, R.C., Patterson, H.R., and Peacock, E. (1974). Referrals to hospitals in an East Midlands city — a medical audit. *Journal of the Royal College of General Practitioners* **24**, 304–19.

Fry, J. (1972). Twenty-one years of general practice — changing patterns. *Journal of the Royal College of General Practitioners* **22**, 521–8.

Gillam, D.M. (1985). Referral to consultants — the National Health Service versus private practice. *Journal of the Royal College of General Practitioners* **35**, 15–18.

Jones, D.T. (1987). A survey of hospital outpatient referral rates, Wales 1985. *British Medical Journal* **295**, 734–6.

Journal of the Royal College of General Practitioners (1978). Practice activity analysis 5. Referrals to specialists. *Journal of the Royal College of General Practitioners* 28, 251–2.

Madeley, R.J., Evans, J.R., and Muir, B. (1990). The use of routine referral data in the development of clinical audit and management in North Lincolnshire. *Journal of Public Health Medicine* **12**, 1, 22–7.

Marsh, G.N. and McNay, R.A. (1974). Factors affecting work load in general practice — II. *British Medical Journal* **1**, 319–21.

McCormick, A. and Rosenbaum, M. (1990). *Morbidity statistics from general practice 1981–82. Third national study: socio-economic analyses.* HMSO, London.

Moore, A.T. and Roland, M.O. (1989). How much variation in referral rates among general practitioners is due to chance? *British Medical Journal* **298**, 500–2.

Morrell, D.C., Gage, H.G., and Robinson, N.A. (1971). Referral to hospital by general practitioners. *Journal of the Royal College of General Practitioners* **21**, 77–85.

National Audit Office (1991). *NHS Outpatient Services.* HMSO, London.

Noone, A., Goldacre, M., Coulter, A., and Seagroatt, V. (1989). Do referral rates vary widely between practices and does supply of services affect demand? A study in Milton Keynes and the Oxford region. *Journal of the Royal College of General Practitioners* **39**, 404–7.

Reynolds, G.A., Chitnis, J.G., and Roland, M.O. (1991). General practitioner outpatient referrals: do good doctors refer more patients to hospital? *British Medical Journal* **302**, 1250–1.

Roland, M. and Morris, R. (1988). Are referrals by general practitioners influenced by the availability of consultants? *British Medical Journal* **297**, 599–600.

Ross, A.K., Davis, W.A., Horn, G., and Williams, R. (1983). General practice outpatient referrals in North Staffordshire. *British Medical Journal* **287**, 1439–41.

RCGP/OPCS (1986). *1981–1982 Morbidity statistics from general practice. Third national study.* HMSO, London.

Secretaries of State for Social Services, Wales, Northern Ireland and Scotland (1987). *Promoting better health* (White Paper). HMSO, London.

Secretaries of State for Social Services, Wales, Northern Ireland and Scotland (1989). *Working for patients* (White Paper). HMSO, London.

Scott, R. and Gilmore, M. (1966). Studies of hospital outpatient services: 1 The Edinburgh hospitals. *Problems and Progress in Medical Care* (ed. G. McLachlan), pp. 3–41. Oxford University Press, Oxford.

Starey, C.J.H. (1961). A hospital outpatient referral survey: a study of the referral habits of a group of general practitioners. *Journal of the Royal College of General Practice* **4**, 214–22.

Wilkin, D. and Dornan, C. (1990). *General practitioner referrals to hospital. A review of research and its implications for policy and practice.* Centre for Primary Care Research, University of Manchester.

Wilkin, D., Hallam, Leavey, Metcalfe (1987). *Anatomy of urban general practice.* Tavistock, London.

Wilkin, D. and Smith, T. (1986). *Variations in GP referrals to consultants.* Centre for Primary Care Research, University of Manchester.

Wilkin, D. and Smith, A.G. (1987a). Variation in general practitioners' referral rates to consultants. *Journal of the Royal College of General Practitioners* **37**, 350–3.

Wilkin, D. and Smith, T. (1987b). Explaining variation in general practitioner referrals to hospital. *Family Practice* **4** (3), 160–9.

Wilkin, D., Metcalfe, D.H., and Marinker, M. (1989). The meaning of information of GP referral rates to hospitals. *Community Medicine* **11** (1), 65–70.

Wright, H.J. (1968). *General Practice in South West England. Report from general practice 7.* Royal College of General Practitioners.

7 Decision-making and hospital referrals

Roger Jones

Introduction

General practitioners, in contrast to specialists, work in a practice environment in which there is a high prevalence of symptomatic discomfort but a low prevalence of frank disease. This means that they have to employ clinical strategies which are very different to those used in hospital medicine. The GP must, more often than not, diagnose what things are not, rather than what they are, and must make management decisions prior to or instead of diagnostic decisions (Howie 1974). This view is supported by other studies which have suggested that there are real differences between the diagnostic methods of primary care and those of specialist physicians. As an example, family physicians tend to ask fewer history questions and request fewer items of physical examination, but overall ask proportionately more questions about life situations and mental illness (McWhinney 1972; Smith and McWhinney 1975). In another study this notion was challenged, and Barrows *et al.* (1978) found little direct evidence to suggest that the cognitive strategies of the two groups were markedly dissimilar. Simpson *et al.* (1987), using simulated patients, have also reported differences in the amount and nature of diagnostic information collected by family physicians and internists.

The debate was continued by Dixon (1986), who commented on the twin clichés of the specialist as a single-minded biomedical scientist and the family physician as the simple humanist who prefers action to words. He pointed out that, if there is indeed a difference between the cognitive styles of family physicians and specialists, it is less a question of their nature than of the environment in which they are nurtured. It is likely to be the domain of the problem that places demands on problem solvers and determines the skills they need, even though there may be some element of self-selection in people who do or do not enjoy working in a particular field. If problem-solving is a process which is adaptive to the way people think, it would be surprising if it were not also adaptable to what they have to think about.

The referral decision made by an individual clinician lies at the heart of any attempt to understand the referral process or to explain the wide variations which exist amongst GPs in their rates of hospital referral.

Clinical decision-making has been a subject of intense research interest and activity for over 20 years and has provided many insights into the ways in which we arrive at diagnoses and management plans in clinical practice. More recently, attempts have been made to develop decision-making theories to provide an explanatory framework for the referral decision, although at present no comprehensive explanatory model has been developed, still less one capable of predicting referral behaviour.

Clinical decision-making

The study of clinical decision-making falls broadly into two distinct areas of activity. Firstly, *decision analysis* is based upon a rigorous, mathematical approach to the collection and evaluation of evidence and the clinical actions following from this, using Bayesian theories of prior probabilities and incorporating other objective descriptions of the consequences of clinical decisions, such as expected utility analysis. This approach to the study of clinical decision-making often involves the use of decision trees and algorithms and is generally aimed at charting a rational course through a diagnostic and therapeutic maze, from which outcomes are judged on the basis of their clinical efficacy and cost-effectiveness. Decision analysis incorporates information obtained from application of the principles of clinical epidemiology and the results of randomized controlled trials, so that consensus views about management of specific clinical problems can be achieved.

The second approach to the study of clinical decision making can, broadly, be described as *'psychological'*. Using research methodologies derived from cognitive psychology, investigators seek to analyse the thought processes occurring in the mind of the decision maker in an attempt to provide a description of the cognitive events leading to a clinical decision. These include the ways in which clinical and other information is collected by the decision maker, diagnostic hypotheses are generated, reviewed, and refined, and clinical information is stored and accessed in the decision-maker's mind. Much decision-making work of this kind has depended upon a technique known as video-stimulated recall, in which real or simulated consultations are video-taped and played back to the physician, who is asked at frequent intervals about the diagnostic thinking leading to the formulation, generally, of a clinical diagnosis.

Following early decision-making research in North America in the 1970s, recent interest has focused on the differences in decision-making between novices and experts and between generalists and specialists, as well as in the ways in which we store clinical information and use our knowledge to make decisions. The emphasis in much of this research has been on diagnosis rather than management, and only recently has work of this kind been applied to the referral decision.

Both of these approaches to the study of decision making are valuable, but until recently clinical decision-making has been studied as if it is a detached and entirely objective activity, into which the emotional context in which the decision is made is not allowed to intrude. This is clearly inappropriate, and attempts are now being made to integrate the emotional component of decision-making into the more traditional model.

This chapter describes in more detail both clinical decision analysis and the cognitive psychological approach to decision-making theory, and examines the ways in which they can be applied to the referral decision. As many questions as answers are generated by doing this, but these uncertainties form the basis for important research questions and future studies which are needed to advance our understanding of the complexities of outpatient referral decisions.

Clinical decision analysis

There is no doubt that clinical decision analysis aims to provide guidance for clinicians without regard to subjective or emotional considerations. Clinical decision analysis is a formal method for decision-making which takes into account the likelihood of the outcomes of actions, the risks and benefits associated with these outcomes, and value judgments on how the patients' interests are best to be served (Pauker and Kassirer 1987).

Although much of the work on clinical decision analysis has been undertaken in the secondary care setting, the reasons for which an objective approach to clinical decision-making is required are common to the work of generalist and specialist physicians. We all work in conditions of clinical uncertainty and frequently have to make decisions on the basis of incomplete information. In the hospital setting clinicians frequently have difficulty in interpreting diagnostic tests and processing clinical information derived from them. In general practice we tend to use the clinical history rather than laboratory investigations to make our initial diagnostic decisions, but are working under similar conditions of uncertainty. There is good evidence too that all physicians, experts and novices, specialists and generalists, possess a number of clinical biases which can interfere with rational decision-making. These include inaccurate estimates of the prevalence of common diseases, difficulties of salience bias, in which decision making is affected by the characteristics and outcomes experienced in recently-seen patients, and a phenomenon known an 'anchoring', in which an initial judgment is held more strongly than subsequent clinical information should permit (Tversky and Kahneman 1972).

In order to give objectivity to the processing of clinical information, clinical decision analysis has been developed and is assembled from three simple building blocks (Balla *et al.* 1989). The first of these is the use of 2×2 tables used to help visualize statistical properties of test results.

The sensitivity (the true positive rate) and specificity (the true negative rate) can be presented in such tables, so that the predictive value of test results can be calculated (Sackett *et al.* 1985). Secondly, Bayes' theorem permits the calculation both of the probability of the presence of the condition given certain clinical findings and the revision of the probabilities associated with any given test results (Balla *et al.* 1975). As an example, Bayes' theorem allows an estimation of the probability of acute appendicitis being present when there is pain in the right iliac fossa, associated with tenderness and guarding in a 21-year-old woman. Thirdly, decision trees can be used to provide an explicit, pictorial representation of alternative management strategies. They can incorporate probabilities and utility assessments into the management options available to the clinician, and sensitivity analysis to answer 'What if' questions can be performed by changing the values of variables in the tree.

These 'mathematical' approaches are, clearly, more applicable to patients receiving care in the hospital setting, in which the evaluation of test results and decisions about treatment can be more accurately incorporated into a decision tree. As an example, a decision tree can be constructed to help determine whether medical or surgical treatment is used in a patient suffering a transient ischaemic attack; an estimate of the probability of the various possible outcomes — recovery, stroke, or death — is incorporated to generate the expected value for each strategy. Clinical decision analysis, on the other hand, can form the basis of management strategies in general practice, assuming that the basic clinical information about the condition in question is available. Unfortunately this is often not the case; clear descriptions of the natural history and outcomes of therapy of many of the common conditions which we see in our surgeries are often not available, so that much management in general practice is empirical and, in addition, suffers from some of the biases mentioned above.

Even in the hospital setting, clinical decision analysis is not a widely accepted component of routine clinical care. Clinicians remain reluctant to use probability-based estimates, even though they may intuitively be aware that diagnosis and management are based on such terms as 'very likely' or 'not very likely', preferring these terms to more precise statements involving numerical probabilities. In clinical decision-making, very small probabilities are often over-weighted, so that rare events can loom larger psychologically than they would in a decision analysis of the problem. As a result of this, decision analysis can lead to results which, though consistent with the information supplied and with the rules of combining various estimates, 'feel wrong' psychologically. As an example, if we have recently seen a rare side-effect of a certain therapy, although the odds on a particular patient running into trouble are not increased, we may still resist 'mathematical' reassurance. Or if we had recently 'failed' to refer a young patient with rectal bleeding who turned out to have cancer, our response to the next patient with rectal bleeding is likely to be at odds with the 'correct' course of action. Many clinicians also feel uncomfortable when asked to attach numerical values to outcomes, so that the use of decision analysis to determine 'utility' is resisted, partly because it may lead to providing overprecise ways of measuring outcomes which may appear to be, or may well be, immeasurable.

Expected utility theory, which is a standard method used to predict people's choices under uncertainty, is also under review (Hellinger 1989). It is clear that when faced with uncertain choices related to health outcomes, many of us are risk-averse in our decision-making; rather than regarding the decision making process as an objective exercise, research is beginning to draw parallels between decision-making and gambling. There appears to be significant variability between the risk attitudes of individuals for any given gamble and significant variability in the risk attitudes of a given individual across different gambles. This variability of risk attitudes suggests that these are not absolute but are functions of the parameters of the gamble; in other words, they depend on our perception of what is at stake.

In summary, it seems unlikely that classical clinical decision analysis will form an important part of the explicit decision-making process in primary care, and certainly does not help us to understand the ways in which we make referral decisions. However, its importance lies in its ability to determine, given some of the reservations mentioned here, the likely outcomes of different courses of action in the management of clinical problems and, when the clinical information is sufficient, may form a useful approach to the construction of management guidelines and protocols for common conditions. This would clearly have an impact on referral decision-making, particularly if it can be shown that the timing and circumstances of certain referrals were linked to improvements or deteriorations in clinical outcomes. One example of this might be the investigation of patients with upper abdominal pain. Although it can be argued that, in patients at low risk of upper gastrointestinal malignancy, early investigation is inappropriate, there is evidence that in patients with non-ulcer dyspepsia, following a negative endoscopy rates of consultation and prescribing fall substantially (Jones 1988). Early referral in selected patients might, therefore, be associated with improved outcomes both in terms of resource utilization and health status. Little information of this kind is currently available, but clinical decision analysis clearly has a potential role in the evaluation of alternative referral strategies for common conditions.

It is perhaps appropriate to emphasize here that clinical decision analysis deserves inclusion in undergraduate curricula and in continuing medical education. By doing so, defects in 'intuitive' decision-making can be identified, fundamental gaps in our knowledge of the natural history of common conditions can be pointed out, concepts such as risks, costs, benefits, and utilities can be introduced into clinical reasoning, and an explicit and open approach to problem-solving can be engendered.

Computer-assisted decision-making

Because of the mathematical basis of clinical decision analysis, the utilization of computer technology to calculate diagnostic odds and utilities was a natural next step. This approach has been used with some success in, for example, the computer-aided diagnosis of abdominal pain, where more accurate selection of patients with suspected appendicitis for surgery has led to savings in terms of hospital bed utilization (Adams *et al.* 1986). A computer-aided diagnostic system for dyspepsia has also been developed, and although it is capable of generating a useful, hierarchical list of diagnostic probabilities, has been shown to have poor transferability from one demographic area to another (Knill-Jones *et al.* 1985; Linberg *et al.* 1987). Systems of this kind generally involve the completion, at a keyboard, of fairly detailed questionnaires by the clinician, and none of them are as yet sufficiently robust or compact for use in the general practice setting, and are not likely to have an impact on referral decision-making for the foreseeable future.

Decision-making theory

In the early 1970s Elstein's group from Michigan began to publish a series of studies based on video-stimulated recall of simulated consultations. From this work emerged the hypothetico–deductive theory of clinical decision-making (Elstein *et al.* 1978). According to this, the clinician generates a number of hypotheses either simultaneously or rapidly sequentially very early in the clinical encounter. Between three and six hypotheses are initially held, some of which may have been generated on the basis of the doctor's previous knowledge of the patient, rather than on an awareness of the presenting complaint. Following this, the physician begins to collect information, using 'search and scan strategies' and 'cue interpretation', constantly redefining and refining the hypotheses, discarding those that do not fit the clinical information obtained from the history and examination, and focusing more closely on the problem formulation for making subsequent decisions about diagnosis and management.

This model of clinical decision-making has been widely accepted for many years, but is now recognized to suffer from a number of limitations (McGuire 1984). Like clinical decision analysis, the hypothetico–deductive model does not readily accommodate the emotional context in which decisions are made, and provides a poor explanatory model for the wide differences which exist between physicians in their diagnostic and management decisions, including referral decisions. There is also accumulating evidence which suggests that other cognitive processes are at work in the mind of the decision maker, which do not fit the hypothetico–deductive model particularly well.

One of the first inconsistencies is concerned with the acquisition of clinical data against which the working hypotheses are considered and either discarded or developed. A number of early studies on decision making related the amount of clinical information gathered and the subsequent length of the decision chain to the experience or otherwise of the problem-solver in a commonsense way (Kleinmutz 1968). In a more recent study it was shown that GPs varied widely in the amount of information required to solve management problems in a series of simulated consultations. There was no correlation between the professional experience of the doctors in this study and the amount or nature of data collected; there was consistency within subjects, but not within problems, in the amount of information required for problem-solving. This suggests that individual clinicians possess unique and complex knowledge bases and, consequently, require different amounts and kinds of information for problem-solving (Jones 1987). These findings are not necessarily in conflict with the hypothetico–deductive model — doctors may simply use the model in different ways — but serve as a reminder that the individual clinician is at the centre of the reasoning process and that the intellectual and emotional context in which decisions are made will be different for each of us.

A number of other studies have cast more serious doubt upon the hypothetico–deductive model. In an important review McGuire (1984) commented that subjects in such experiments are frequently asked merely to label something, rather than to solve a problem. Very general theories about decision-making have been generated by studies on very small numbers of subjects and tasks. In a review of the evidence supporting the hypothetico–deductive model Groen and Patel (1985) have cast doubt on whether this method is really used in medical problem-solving at all. It may be, for example, that experts, as opposed to novices, use 'strong' problem-solving methods which depend on complex knowledge bases held by individual doctors, implying that an element of pattern recognition is perhaps of greater importance than has previously been accepted. This idea has also been developed by Bordage and Zacks (1984) who have evolved the concept of prototype matching, a refinement of pattern-recognition, in which the decision maker considers to what extent the problem presented to him is 'prototypic' of a group of disorders of which he possesses a knowledge base. A similar notion has been developed by Gale and Marsden (1983), who have evolved the concept of 'forceful features'. They found that a number of thinking processes were common to all medical problem-solvers, irrespective of their experience, but that

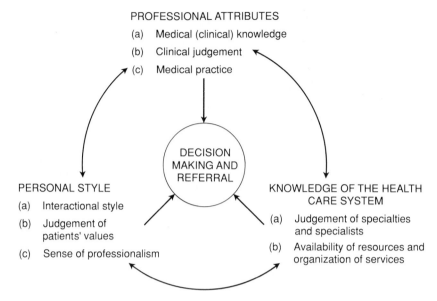

Fig. 7.1 Framework of referral decision making. (Dowie 1983)

the content of thought may be different in each case. Gale and Marsden's 'forceful features' represent aspects of a given clinical problem, specific to each individual problem-solver, which act as triggers for accessing long-term memory. Finally, one other criticism of the video-stimulated recall methods of Elstein's group is that their subjects may well have been giving an account not of what they did, but rather a reconstruction of how they thought the problem should have been solved.

The referral decision

The first real breakthrough in understanding the nature of the referral decision came from an important study of outpatient referrals conducted by Dowie (1983). Interview material collected in this work suggested that a substantial part of the reason for the variability in family doctors' referral rates lay in their cognitive processes — differing confidence in their clinical judgement and differing awareness of the base rate probabilities of the occurrence of life-threatening events. These interviews also suggested that GPs had differing current states of medical knowledge, hence their variable reliance on information provided by certain investigations. Dowie also found that GPs are keen to sustain their esteem in the eyes of their consultant colleagues. She attempted to synthesize these elements into a model of the referral decision itself, placing this at the centre of the framework of referral decision-making (Fig. 7.1).

Table 7.1 *Effective decision-making (Janis and Mann 1977)*

The decision-maker, to the best of his ability and within his information-processing capabilities:

(1) thoroughly canvasses alternative courses of action;
(2) surveys the full range of objectives;
(3) carefully weighs the costs and risks of negative consequences;
(4) intensively searches for new information;
(5) correctly assimilates all new information;
(6) re-examines the positive and negative consequences of all known alternatives;
(7) makes detailed provisions for implementing or executing the chosen course of action, with contingency plans if various known risks were to materialize.

In order to construct this model, Dowie drew on the Conflict Theory of Janis and Mann (1977), who see man not as a rational calculator, always ready to work out the best solution, but as a warm-blooded mammal and a reluctant decision-maker 'beset by conflict, doubts and worry, struggling with incongruous longings, antipathies and loyalties and seeking relief by procrastinating, rationalising or denying responsibility for his own choices'. Janis and Mann concluded that for decision-making procedures to be of high quality, seven major criteria must be fulfilled. These are shown in Table 7.1. Janis and Mann also recognized the importance of the emotional context in which the decision is made, and this was also incorporated into Dowie's model. Five coping patterns may be adopted in situations generating psychological stress, such as decisional conflict, and these are as follows:

(1) unconflicted inertia;

(2) unconflicted change to a new course of action;

(3) defensive avoidance;

(4) hyper-vigilance;

(5) vigilance.

When an individual is faced with a decision of consequence and experiences very little conflict or stress, he or she is unlikely to give the decision much thought or to seek out new information, and will adopt the strategies of 'unconflicted inertia' or 'unconflicted change'. On the other hand, if stress is very intense it is likely to give rise to 'defensive avoid-ance' or 'hyper-vigilance'. In other words, when the decision maker is under no stress at all, throwaway decisions of poor quality may be made; if the level of stress is intolerably high, equally bad decision-making may result. It is only when the decision maker is under moderate stress that he/she is best able to process information in a vigilant fashion.

Dowie developed a model of the referral decision (Fig. 7.2) in which Janis and Mann's Conflict Theory has been modified to represent the stages in reaching this decision. Although much of her transcripted interview material 'fits' with this model, Dowie concedes that whether these specific examples were in any way typical of the doctor's decision-making style, over time, is unknown. Similarly, the reasons why some GPs more frequently exit from this model by referring their patients than other doctors are obscure, and Dowie's data are insufficiently comprehensive to draw any firm conclusions about this. She did, however, offer suggestions for defects in clinical reasoning which might be associated with variations in referral rates, including conservatism, a tendency to over-prediction (making statements about diagnostic probabilities or disease outcomes which are not justified by the evidence available — see Elstein 1976), and defective judgements of probabilities when faced with certain symptoms (Tversky and Kahneman 1972).

In an important review of the variation in GP referrals to hospital, Wilkin and Smith (1987) concluded that the causes of variation between GPs in referral rates remains unexplained, and that attempts to account for differing referral rates in terms of both patient characteristics and doctor/practice characteristics have largely been unsuccessful. The suggestion that doctors have unique 'referral thresholds', combining characteristics that might bear on referral habits such as training, experience, tolerance of uncertainty, sense of autonomy, and personal enthusiasm, seems merely to re-state the problem (Cummins *et al.* 1981).

Wilkin and Smith criticized Dowie's model firstly because it emphasized referral in conditions of diagnostic uncertainty to the virtual exclusion of decisions to refer for treatment, secondly because it is a model based on the importance of acute 'serious' conditions, dealing inadequately with chronic and 'non-serious' conditions, and perhaps most importantly because it is based on a model of medical decision-making which regards diagnosis as the central component of the process. This is also a major criticism of the hypothetico–deductive model of clinical decision-making.

GPs frequently make referral decisions for reasons other than diagnosis, and Wilkin and Smith attempted to develop a further explanatory framework as a means to understanding the referral decision and possible sources of variation. They advanced their own model (Fig. 7.3) as a more comprehensive account of the referral decision, framing the initial question in more general terms, rather than emphasizing the importance of diagnosis and, while conceding that diagnostic uncertainty may be important, concentrating on other questions which the GP might feel it necessary to ask in order to determine appropriate action. If the doctor decides that

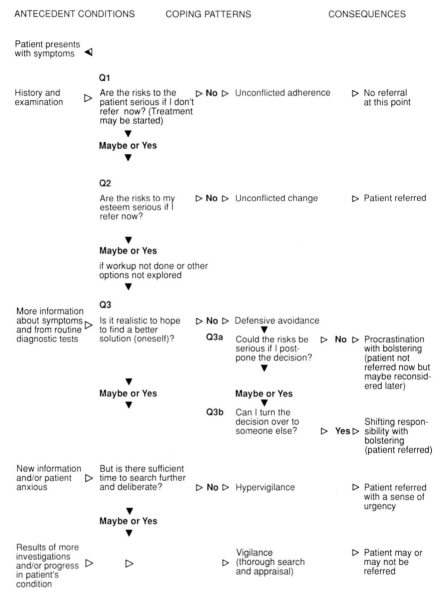

Fig. 7.2 A model of the referral decision. (Dowie 1983)

Reproduced by permission of the King's Fund Centre, and taken from *General practitioners and consultants: A study of outpatient referrals* by Robin Dowie, published by the King's Fund Centre 1983.

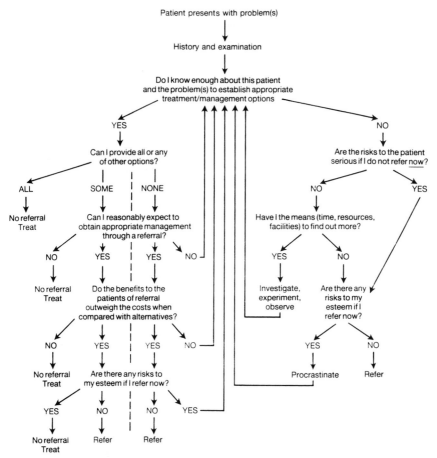

Fig. 7.3 An alternative model of the referral decision. (Wilkin and Smith 1987) Reproduced by permission of Oxford University Press, and taken from Explaining variation in general practitioner referrals to hospital. *Family Practice*, **4**, 160–9.

enough information is available to determine an appropriate course of action, the decision whether or not to refer revolves around judgments of the likelihood of achieving desired results through a referral. The model allows that, in many instances, there will be a variety of management options, some of which the GP will be able to provide and others which will require referral. Thus, for example, for a patient suffering from depression the GP may consider prescribing antidepressant drugs, referral to a psychiatrist, and referral to the social and voluntary agencies.

The attraction of Wilkin and Smith's model is that it is applicable to a wider range of clinical activities than Dowie's, it recognizes that diagnostic uncertainty is only one of a variety of reasons for making a referral, and introduces a number of judgments which are likely to affect the decision. Applying this model to the problem of variation in referral rates, there are clearly a number of points in the referral decision process at which variation is likely to occur and which might explain some of the differences observed amongst GPs.

The importance of the work both of Dowie and of Wilkin and Smith is that it focuses research enquiry firmly on the thought processes of the referring clinician, whilst taking account of the emotional context in which the referral decision is made. Implicit in these approaches is the belief that referral decision-making is not mysterious and immutable, but is something susceptible to examination and rational explanation.

The referral decision and the future

The fact that, by definition, a number of GPs make clinical decisions at the extremes of variation has not been lost on administrators and those responsible for resource management. There is a strong and clear tendency to regard GPs whose rates of referral, investigation or prescribing fall outside an arbitrary norm as aberrant and wasteful. Yet we know so little about the consequences of high and low referral rates, in terms of resource utilization, quality of life, and health status of patients and other variables in the health equation. It is clearly premature to make judgements about 'good' and 'bad' practice in relation to simple measurement of referral rates.

The importance of decision-making research in relation to referral is that the explanatory models generated embrace many factors which traditionally fall outside the 'rational' model of medical behaviour. Foremost of these is uncertainty, which may operate on at least three levels. Firstly, there may be genuine, shared uncertainty about the natural history of common conditions seen in general practice. Much of our therapeutic guidance derives from studies of disease performed in a secondary care setting, and we need more information about the natural history of the common conditions which form the basis of our daily work. Secondly, the decision maker may experience uncertainty in relation to the current state of medical knowledge; he or she may be out-of-date or unfamiliar with certain areas of medicine and require further information in order to make management decisions. Thirdly, and perhaps most importantly, there may be real problems with toleration of diagnostic uncertainty in the mind of the decision maker with some doctors needing clear answers early in the course of an illness, while others are content to temporize, to use time as a therapeutic tool and to await developments. The individual contributions of these dimensions of uncertainty are not known, but there are suggestions from decision-making research that they play a part in determining some of our clinical behaviour (Jones 1990). Much of our medical education teaches us that we should be decisive and confident, and much inappropriate 'certainty' is probably generated by this traditional medical posture. But indecisiveness and uncertainty are not the same thing — indecision in the face of utter certainty is commonplace, while it is possible to be quite clear about the next steps in management under conditions of considerable diagnostic uncertainty.

Also implicit in the models of decision-making proposed by Dowie and by Wilkin and Smith is the acceptance that the environment in which the decision is made is important. At its most basic this may represent the pressure of time experienced during a surgery by a GP, but may have more subtle connotations, including the professional support individual GPs enjoy from their colleagues, both in general practice and hospital medicine, the working environment of the practice itself, the extent to which ancillary and nursing staff are provided to participate in team care, the premises and locality in which the practice is situated, and, beyond that, the family and personal relationships and stresses experienced by the doctor on a given occasion. The problem of stress in the GP is attracting increasing research interest, as we begin to look more and more critically at the traditional model of personal family medicine and its possible links with the quality of care which we are able to provide (Winefield and Anstey 1990).

Conclusion

Future research into the referral decision needs to engage all of these problems and has to aim not only at providing us with guidance on which we can based an appraisal of our own referral behaviour but, more importantly than that, discuss in a non-threatening and non-judgmental way the referral patterns of our colleagues, which may be very different from our own. Until information of this kind and depth is available, we make superficial judgements linking quality of care and referral rates at our peril.

References

Adams, I.D. *et al.* (1986). *British Medical Journal* **293**, 800–4.
Balla, J.I., Iansek, R., and Elstein, A. (1975). Bayesian diagnosis in presence of pre-existing disease. *Lancet* **1**, 326–9.
Balla, J.I., Elstein, A.S., and Christensen, C. (1989). Obstacles to acceptance of clinical decision analysis. *British Medical Journal* **298**, 579–82.
Barrows, H.S., Feightner, J.W., Neufeld, V.R., and Norman, G.R. (1978). Analysis of the clinical methods of medical students and physicians. *Final report submitted to the Province of Ontario Department of Health and Physician Services Inc. Foundation* **81**, 187–8.
Bordage, G. and Zacks, R. (1984). The structure of medical knowledge in the

memories of medical students and general practitioners: categories and proto-types. *Medical Education* **18**, 406–16.

Cummins, R.O., Jarman, B., and White, P.M. (1981). Do general practitioners have different 'referral thresholds'? *British Medical Journal* **282**, 1037–9.

Dixon, A.S. (1986). 'There's a lot of it about': clinical strategies in family practice. *Journal of the Royal College of General Practitioners* **36**, 468–71.

Dowie, R. (1983). *General practitioners and consultants: a study of outpatient referrals*. King Edward's Hospital Fund for London, London.

Elstein, A. (1976). Clinical judgement, psychological research and medical practice. *Science* **194**, 696–700.

Elstein, A.S., Shulman, L.S., Sprafka, S.S. (1978). *An analysis of clinical reasoning* Harvard University Press, Cambridge, Ma.

Gale, J. and Marsden, P. (1984). *Medical diagnosis from student to clinician*. Oxford University Press, Oxford.

Groen, G.J. and Patel, V.M. (1985). Medical problem-solving; some questionable assumptions. *Medical Education* **19**, 95–9.

Hellinger, F.J. (1989). Expected utility theory and risky choices with health outcomes. *Medical Care* **27**, 273–9.

Howie, J.G.R. (1974). Further observations on diagnosis and management of general practice respiratory illness using simulated patient consultations. *British Medical Journal* **2**, 540–43.

Janis, I.L. and Mann, L. (1977). *Decision making. A psychological analysis of conflict, choice and commitment*. The Free Press, New York.

Jones, R. (1988). What happens to patients with non-ulcer dyspepsia after endoscopy? *Practitioner* **232**, 75–8.

Jones, R.H. (1987). Data collection in decision-making: a study in general practice. *Medical Education* **21**, 99–104.

Jones, R.H. (1990). *Self-care and primary care of dyspepsia*. DM Thesis, University of Southampton.

Knill-Jones, R.P., Dunwoodie, W.M., and Crean, G.P. (1985). A computer-aided diagnostic decision system for dyspepsia. In *Decision making in general practice*. (ed. M. Sheldon, E.J. Brook, and A. Rector). Macmillan, London. pp. 203–20.

Kleinmutz, B. (1968) The processing of clinical information by man and machine. In *The formal representation of human judgement* (ed. B. Kleinmutz). Wiley, New York. pp. 149–86.

Lindberg, G., Seensalu, R., Nilsson, L.H., Forsell, P., Kager, L., and Knill-Jones, R.P. (1987). Transferability of a computer system for medical history taking and decision support in dyspepsia. A comparison of indicants for peptic ulcer disease. *Scandinavian Journal of Gastroenterology* Suppl **128**, 190–9.

McGuire, C. (1984). Medical problem solving — a critique of the literature. In *Proceedings of the Twenty Third Annual Conference*. Association of American Medical Colleges, San Francisco.

McWhinney, I.R. (1972). Problem-solving and decision-making in primary medical practice. *Proceedings of the Royal Society of Medicine* **65**, 35–8.

Pauker, S.G. and Kassirer, J.P. (1987). Decision analysis. *New England Journal of Medicine* **316**, 250–8.

Sackett, D.L., Haynes, R.B., and Tugwell, P. (1985). *Clinical epidemiology: a basic science for clinical medicine*. Little, Brown and Company, Boston.

Simpson, D.E. *et al.* (1987). The diagnostic process in primary care: a comparison of general internists and specialists. *Social Science and Medicine* **25**, 861–6.

Smith, D.H. and McWhinney, I.R. (1975). Comparison of the diagnostic methods of family physicians and internists. *Journal of Medical Education* **50**, 264–70.

Tversky, A. and Kahneman, D. (1972). Judgement under uncertainty: heuristics and biases. In *Judgement under uncertainty, heuristics and biases* (ed. D. Kahneman, P. Slovic, and A. Tversky). Cambridge University Press. Cambridge.

Wilkin, D. and Smith, A. (1987). Explaining variation in general practitioner referrals to hospital. *Family Practice* **4**, 160–9.

Winefield, H.R. and Anstey, T.J. (1990). Job stress in general practice: practitioner age, sex and attitudes as predictors. *Family Practice* **8**, 140–4.

8 Communication between GPs and specialists

Martin Roland

Introduction

The clear division of the NHS into primary and secondary care means that, apart from self-referral to casualty departments and a small number of direct access clinics, there is usually an exchange of information between GP and specialist when a patient is seen at hospital. The GP writes a letter when he or she refers a patient and the outpatient referral is followed by a letter from the specialist once the patient has been seen. An inpatient admission is often followed by a discharge note written on the day of discharge or a few days later, with a fuller typed summary following some time later. Telephone communication between GPs and specialists about outpatient referrals and hospital discharges is comparatively uncommon. In this chapter some of the weaknesses of these traditional methods of communication between GPs and specialists are reviewed. Developments of the basic model of communication are reviewed, including shuttle records, patient-held records, and electronic communication using 'smart cards'. Finally, the role of the 1991 reforms of the NHS will be discussed in the light of their far-reaching potential for altering the nature of communication between GPs and consultants.

There is a considerable literature on the deficiencies of communication between GPs and consultants, and it is concentrated on certain areas, in particular discharge summaries, drug information in letters, and psychiatric referrals. In reviewing the published literature it is important to realize that there is likely to be substantial publication bias. Research is likely to have been carried out in geographical locations where there is local dissatisfaction with communication, and in specialties where there are particular problems with communication. It may be unjustified therefore to extrapolate from data in published papers to communication between GPs and consultants in general, and to assume either that all GPs' letters are inadequate or that no consultants send prompt summaries on their patients. However, the unsatisfactory areas identified in the literature can be used to highlight areas which can be used to identify appropriate standards for communication between doctors, and therefore used as a basis for audit.

Referral letters from GPs to specialists

The first systematic study of referral letters was published by De Alarcon and Hodson in 1964. They surveyed 500 letters to a London teaching hospital and found that 88 per cent were handwritten, only 23 per cent mentioned the patients' drug treatment, clinical findings were only mentioned in 22 per cent of letters, and past medical history in only 11 per cent. Despite this, perhaps surprisingly, only 2 per cent of letters fell into the infamous category of simply saying 'Please see and treat'. The unacceptably brief letter has, however, assumed a disproportionately important place in the folklore of referrals partly because, as De Alarcon notes, negative feelings aroused by bad letters disturb objectivity.

General practice has been transformed since 1964 and standards of communication have improved in many respects. Referral letters are more frequently typed; 76 per cent of a series of 628 referrals to a Doncaster orthopaedic clinic were typed (M. Roland, personal communication), as were virtually all of a series of 600 referrals including urgent referrals to 6 clinics in Cambridge (A. Fertig, personal communication). However, letters may still be brief; in a study of 288 orthopaedic referrals to Nottingham hospitals only 27 per cent included any past medical history and only 27 per cent listed current medication (Jacobs and Pringle 1990), and only 39.5 per cent of 144 letters to four medical clinics written by Dutch GPs were judged 'good' or 'excellent' by an independent panel of GPs and specialists (Westerman *et al.* 1990). In a series of 306 referral letters for hypertension (Juncosa *et al.* 1990) letters from doctors practising in health centres were more likely to be detailed, and more likely to meet a set of standards for referral of hypertension. These authors reported only one letter which simply read 'Hypertension, please see'.

It is difficult to form judgements about whether referral letters are 'good' or 'bad' without considering what they ought to contain, not least because individual specialists and GPs may make different judgements about the same letter (Westerman *et al.* 1990). It is readily apparent that the information which needs to be in a referral letter will depend both on the specialty and the particular type of problem which is to be referred, so it is worth considering what information specialists say they would like to receive.

What information should referral letters contain?

Details of the patient's medication has been judged by specialists to be the most important item of information in the referral letter in three studies (Long and Atkins 1974; Williams and Wallace 1974; Pullen and Yellowlees 1985). Criticism of the accuracy of drug information in referral letters has been made in relation to geriatric referrals (Gilchrist *et al.* 1987) and ophthalmology admissions (Claoué and Elkington 1986), and it would be difficult to contest the idea that GPs should include accurate drug information in their letters. The fact that these two critical papers are from geriatric and ophthalmology departments is not surprising as patients in these specialties are often elderly and may be unclear about their own medication. Furthermore, the problem is not confined to GPs; in a study of general medical outpatients, both GPs and hospital doctors appeared to be unaware of some important drugs which patients were taking (Price *et al.* 1986).

Other items considered important in a referral letter are likely to be more specialty specific. In the study carried out by Williams and Wallace psychiatrists rated legibility of the letter and past psychiatric history as the most important items after details of medication; details of the present complaint were considered less important, presumably because the psychiatrist expected to obtain those details him or herself. Psychiatrists in an Edinburgh study preferred their letters to be about a page in length, with headings for separate sections (Blaney and Pullen 1989).

It might seem self-evident that the reason for referral should be contained in a referral letter, particularly as GPs' and specialists' perceptions about the reason for a referral may not always match (Grace and Armstrong 1987; Doeleman 1987). However, this is an area about which GPs feel sensitive. Some GPs in Dowie's (1983) study commented that they thought it would be presumptuous to imply to the specialist that he or she was expected to carry out a particular diagnostic or therapeutic procedure. Due respect and tact for the specialist should not preclude the GP from explaining the reasons for the referral, especially as his agenda may not be the same as the patient's (Grace and Armstrong 1987). While the reason for referral may be obvious — for example, for diagnosis or for a particular therapeutic procedure — other reasons may be less obvious. It may be that a relative is exerting pressure on the GP to refer, or that the GP or the patient needs to have rare organic disease ruled out before they can proceed with the management of the patient's psychosomatic symptoms. Since the referral letter is by far the commonest method by which GPs communicate with specialists, it would be completely unproductive if letters did not help specialists to understand the problems faced by their colleagues in primary care. In this context, it is interesting to note that letters written to named consultants tend to be of a higher quality than those simply sent to a named specialty (Long and Atkins 1974) and letters to named consultants are associated with more informative replies (Jacob and Pringle 1990). Wilkin and Smith (1987) have emphasized that a decision to refer to a specialist involves consideration of possible loss of face by the GP. This may well explain why fuller letters are written to named consultants and it emphasizes that the referral is part of a live relationship between GPs and consultants. However, in a study critical of the standard of referral letters for patients requiring urgent assessment, letters from deputizing doctors were found to contain clearer information than those from GPs (Morrison and Pennycook 1991).

When referring a patient the GP should consider the following as items of information which may be useful for the specialist:

(1) presenting problem;

(2) history of presenting problem;

(3) examination findings;

(4) current drug treatment;

(5) allergies;

(6) past treatment of presenting problem;

(7) past medical history;

(8) social circumstances;

(9) results of investigations;

(10) reason for referral;

(11) expectation of follow-up;

(12) urgency of referral.

It will often not be relevant to include information on all these items, and the information required will vary between specialties. In almost all referrals it will be relevant to include details of the presenting problem and the reason for referral unless it is implicit in the rest of the letter. Details of current drug treatment and past treatment for the presenting problem should always be in the letter. The importance of examination findings, past medical history, social history, and results of investigations will vary from referral to referral. Past medical and psychiatric history and past treatment of the problem would be essential parts of a psychiatric referral, but might not be relevant for a dermatology referral. The GP's expectation of follow-up will sometimes be relevant when a patient is being referred with a chronic disease; it may not be clear to the specialist whether he is being asked to provide a one-off opinion or to help with the ongoing management of the patient. Because the requirements of a letter inevitably depend on the problem being referred, scoring systems for letters, which score a letter depending on the presence or absence of certain items of information, should be used with some caution.

In a recent survey of consultants' opinions on what should be in GPs' letters (Newton *et al.* 1992) over 90 per cent of consultants thought that a statement of the problem, the reason for referral, and current medication were 'always' or 'usually' important. These three items were rated of greatest importance by the consultants, followed by past medical history, the GP's expectations of the referral, and examination findings.

Specialists' letters to GPs

The major criticism levelled at letters, discharge notes, and discharge summaries is that they may fail to arrive altogether. In reviewing these papers it is again important to consider publication bias which is likely to lead to selective over-investigation and over-reporting of unsatisfactory situations. Nevertheless, some of the results are alarming; for example, 24 per cent of letters about referrals never being received (McGlade *et al.* 1988), 25 per cent of discharge summaries never being received (Penny 1988), and 53 per cent of patients contacting their GP before any communication had been received (Mageean 1986). A spot survey by Penny showed that on one day 5 per cent of the annual load of discharge summaries (1080 summaries) were waiting to be typed in the hospital, emphasizing that shortage of secretarial resources may be an important factor delaying communication between specialists and GPs. Secretarial shortages were also blamed for a 6–7 week delay in letters being sent from gastroenterology and neurology outpatient clinics in Amsterdam (Westerman *et al.* 1990).

Sandler and Mitchell (1987) compared the relative efficiency of posting the interim discharge summary from a Nottingham hospital or giving it to the patient to deliver to his GP. The GP received 97 per cent of summaries in both groups, but they arrived significantly faster when delivered by patients, with 55 per cent of summaries delivered by hand arriving within one day of the patient's discharge.

What information do GPs want in discharge summaries and clinic letters?

The specialist should consider the following items of information as being of potential value to the patient's GP following an outpatient referral or an admission:

(1) summary of symptoms;

(2) examination findings;

(3) results of investigations;

(4) diagnosis/summary of problem;

(5) management plan;

(6) nature and quantity of drugs issued;

(7) information given to patient/relative;

(8) follow-up arrangement;

(9) advice on future management.

However, the type of information needed by GPs will again depend on the specialty under consideration; for example, in a study of oncology patients (Bado and Williams 1984) the items judged most important were diagnosis, stage of disease, drugs used, and information and prognosis given to the patient, whereas in a study of orthopaedics (Pater and Chapple 1985) drug treatment and details of suggested aftercare were the two items rated most important by the GPs. In two studies of letters from a range of specialties, important details most frequently missing from letters were drug treatment, drug reactions, results of investigations, information given to patients, and details of follow-up plans (Tulloch *et al.* 1975; Harding 1987). In Westerman's study of Dutch specialists and GPs only half of the specialists' letters were judged to be of educational value by an independent panel (Westerman *et al.* 1990), though there was no measure of how frequently educational information for the GP might have been expected to be included. Jacobs and Pringle (1990) also noted missed educational opportunities in a series of orthopaedic letters; less than half of the questions in GPs' referral letters were answered, and only 26 per cent of letters contained any information judged to be of educational value.

In a recent study of the views of Newcastle GPs on what should be in consultants' letters (Newton *et al.* 1992) more than 90 per cent thought that an appraisal of the problem, examination findings, a management plan and an indication of who saw the patient were 'always' or 'usually' important. An indication of what the patient or relative was told, investigation findings, and the time until follow-up were rated as 'always' or 'usually' important by 85 per cent of GPs.

While letters and discharge summaries from most specialties are criticized for the information they omit, those from psychiatrists are sometimes considered too long (Craddock and Craddock 1989). This is probably because the psychiatrists use the discharge summary as an important part of their continuing clinical record, and it therefore may contain more information than that required by the GP.

Communication with nurses

When patients are discharged from hospital following operations communication with community nurses is particularly important. In practice, nurse to nurse communication is often much better than communication from specialist to GP, usually because discharge notes are written more promptly. A delay in sending out a hospital discharge note is a particular problem for those involved in the immediate aftercare of the patient. It is especially important for the primary care team to receive details of the diagnosis, post-operative course (if relevant) and, in the case of malignant disease, what the patient has been told.

Patient-held records

One method of summarizing information about a patient who may be concurrently under the care of a specialist and a GP is for the patient to carry a synopsis of their medical record. This has been employed for many years in obstetrics (the 'co-operation card'), with more recent experiments in which women have been responsible for looking after their entire obstetric record (Zander *et al.* 1978; Draper *et al.* 1986). Patient-held record summaries have also been used for patients with rheumatological conditions (Beyer *et al.* 1985), for diabetics (Hill 1976), and for hypertensive patients (Ezedum and Kerr 1977). This type of record is particularly suitable where frequent changes in the patient's treatment may be needed or where the results of recent examination or investigation need to be known.

In many parts of the country, parents hold a summary of their child's health record, and it has been recommended that there should be a national child health record for child health surveillance (Health Visitors Association *et al.* 1990). A parent-held record is particularly relevant for children as the GP, health visitor, and hospital doctor may all need access to the same information; for example, details of growth and development. This type of record is popular with those parents, GPs, and health visitors who have experience of using them (Macfarlane and Saffin 1990).

If the patient holds all or part of the record, the question arises as to the use that the patient him or herself may make of the information. A quarter of patients in Draper's study found their record difficult to read or worrying, which raises the question of how the information should be recorded if it is to be used as a method of communicating information to the patient as well as between doctors. Specialists initially found it necessary to censor information from 25 per cent of shared diabetic records (Jones *et al.* 1988), though after review 69 per cent of the censored problems were reinstated. As patients' access to their records becomes a right as a result of recent legislation, doctors are less likely to record information which they do not wish the patient to see, and this may increase the use of either limited or full patient-held records. There is certainly potential for further experimentation with patient-held records either as a means of communicating between doctors, or as a means of communicating with patients.

Improving communication between GPs and specialists

Criticism of letters between GPs and consultants focuses on letters not received and items of information missing from letters. A number of initiatives to improve written communication have been described. The simplest of these is to design a structured letter for use within a particular department. Howard (1986) described a structured geriatric discharge note, designed to take the place of a longer summary, which included pre-printed headings for sections on medical assessment, medication, recommended follow up, need for community support, relatives involved, and unresolved problems. 92 per cent of GPs surveyed thought that this was an improvement on the department's previous letter.

An interesting example of a structured discharge summary is used by Sandler and colleagues in Nottingham (Sandler *et al.* 1989). A three-layered form with non-return carbon paper is used to produce a sheet for the hospital records, a sheet for the GP, and a card for the patient. Not all the information to the GP is copied through on to the patient's card. The GP therefore receives all the information given to the patient, including diagnosis, special instructions, and detailed drug regime, but may in addition receive remarks addressed to him personally.

Improved legibility is achieved by using a ward-based computer to generate a combined discharge note and summary. Dunn and Dale (1986) describe the routine use of such a system in a surgical unit. The system has the advantage that the information is structured, the structure can be changed from time to time simply by re-programming the computer, and data from the summaries can be collated automatically for audit.

One of the disadvantages of highly-structured summaries is that they may make an art form out of brevity. The author has experience of receiving one computerized discharge summary which contained 14 items of correctly recorded administrative data, but with the clinical information reading simply:

Diagnosis	Cholecystitis
Operation	Cholecystectomy
Complications	No complications
Outcome	Patient died

This of course does not mean that a structured format precludes the provision of detailed information, and indeed most GPs would prefer to receive brief, accurate information promptly than a verbose summary some weeks later.

Another advantage of a computer-generated summary is that it allows for the possibility of electronic transfer of the information. Software is rapidly being developed to allow communication between computers in practices and hospital computers, and this is likely to become an increasingly popular method of communication; in one survey in 1989, 90 per cent of GPs were positive about the development of electronic links with hospitals especially for receiving laboratory results, discharge letters, notification of admissions, and for booking outpatient appointments directly (Pringle 1989).

The most sophisticated type of electronic communication is the smart card which is a patient-held card on which substantial amounts of data can be electronically recorded. This can be read by smart-card readers located at GP surgeries, hospitals, pharmacies, or other health care facilities. There has been one major trial of the use of patient held smart cards in the UK (NHS Management Executive 1990). In this trial 8500 patients from 2 general practices and almost all the diabetics in Exmouth, a town of 34 000, were issued with 'care cards', with card readers sited in the practices, all the pharmacies in town, and the two local hospitals. The trial was not an outstanding success. There were hardware problems, both with the cards and card readers, not all patients carried their cards, most consultant teams at the district general hospital saw only a handful of cards during the year, and it was logistically difficult to update cards during an outpatient attendance. Despite these drawbacks most users were enthusiastic about the concept of a smart card, and trying to ensure smooth technological and organizational aspects will be a very important part of future experiments with smart cards.

Telephone communication

Communication between GPs and consultants may also be improved by increasing the opportunities to discuss patients on the telephone. At present GPs and consultants communicate relatively infrequently on the telephone. This is partly because of difficulty in finding the GP or consultant at a convenient time. The times when doctors are most readily found are during fixed surgery or outpatient sessions, when they may not wish to be interrupted by telephone calls. Nevertheless, when communication does occur, it may be valuable. Hartog (1988) found that 27 per cent of requests for endocrinology outpatient appointments could be avoided by a telephone call to the referring GP.

In an attempt to improve telephone access to specialists, four consultant orthopaedic surgeons in Doncaster agreed to provide a regular 30-minute time each day (9.30–10.00 a.m.) when they would be available for telephone consultation (Roland and Bewley 1992). The service, called BONELINE, was found to be valuable by GPs who reported that the telephone call definitely avoided the need for referral in 22 per cent of cases, and possibly avoided referral in a further 23 per cent. However, the service was used infrequently, with an average of only 2.5 calls per week compared to 58 written requests for outpatient referrals per week. Improved advertising of the service or provision at a more convenient time of day might have led to better use. However, it may be that orthopaedic problems are less readily dealt with by phone than endocrinological ones.

On the whole, the results of these two studies suggest that there is scope for further experiments to try to make greater use of telephone communication between GPs and specialists, and to document the effect on referral patterns.

Specialist clinics in GP surgeries

One way in which the relationship between GPs and specialists may be radically changed is for specialists to see patients in GPs' surgeries or health centres rather than in the hospital. This offers the opportunity for a change in the type of relationship between the specialist and the GP. If the two are able to meet to discuss patients, either by both participating in the consultation, or by face to face discussion, this greatly increases the potential educational value of a referral. Although there are many individual examples of specialists doing clinics in practices, the specialists who visit practices most frequently are obstetricians (Zander *et al.* 1978; Hall *et al.* 1985; Thomas *et al.* 1987) and psychiatrists. The experience of psychiatrists in primary care offers particular insights into the different ways that specialists can work in the primary care setting.

Nearly 20 per cent of adult psychiatrists surveyed by Strathdee and Williams (1984) reported that they held clinics in primary care settings. Of these, the majority saw new and old patients during their sessions in what has been described as the 'shifted outpatient model', where specialists' work was similar to that in the outpatient department, but with opportunities for better communication with the GP. Patients seen in such clinics are broadly similar to those seen in hospital outpatient clinics (Browning *et al.* 1987; Brown *et al.* 1988), yet in one study in Nottingham a reduction in psychiatric admissions by 20 per cent was reported (Ferguson 1987). This may partly be due to shifting of other members of the psychiatric team to a primary care base to allow, for example, better supervision of patients on long-term neuroleptics, and by increased use of day hospital facilities. The GPs involved in the Nottingham initiative reported that the quality of clinical care offered to patients was improved (Strathdee 1988).

An alternative model to the 'shifted outpatient clinic', and one which may develop from it, is liaison attachment (Mitchell 1983, 1985). In liaison attachment schemes, the role of the psychiatrist in seeing individual patients is greatly reduced. His main role is to meet with the primary health team to discuss psychiatric problems, to increase the skills and confidence of the primary care team and thereby to enable them to take increased responsibility for psychiatric problems. The liaison psychiatrist may see patients with the GP, but with the two doctors taking equally important parts in the consultation so that the effect is to empower the GP to continue to deal with the patient's problem.

Creed and Marks (1989) argue the case for the liaison attachment model as being a more appropriate and more cost effective way to use specialist skills in primary care. There are certainly examples in other specialties where the role of the specialist may change with time. Endocrinologists, for example, may start by visiting a community diabetic clinic on a regular basis to visit patients, but as the skills of the GPs increase and as their management styles harmonize there may only be a need for infrequent visits from the specialist to discuss particular problems. If specialists are to visit primary care settings, then there are clear opportunities to enable GPs to increase their range of skills and responsibilities, and specialists should therefore do more in primary care settings than simply seeing patients in the same way as in their hospital clinics if these opportunities are to be realized.

The changing relationship between general practitioners and specialists

Apart from examples of close liaison such as the areas described in the previous section, the relationship between GPs and specialists remains somewhat at arm's length, with doctors often communicating with each other by letter over many years without actually meeting. In 1991 the NHS was reorganized so that purchasers and providers of health care were separated, and this may lead to some major changes in communication between doctors working in primary and secondary care. Under the new system, health care is purchased either by DHAs on behalf of their resident population or by fundholding practices on behalf of their registered population. In making such purchasing contracts, fundholding GPs have taken a lead in specifying the type of care which they are purchasing. This has included specification of minimum waiting-times for appointment, waiting-time for operation, and standards relating to discharge summaries. Fundholders seem to be making particular use of the opportunity to invite specialists into their own practices, with some even employing a specialist to see patients or to advise in their surgeries. Some GPs have negotiated for their patients to be put directly on operative waiting-lists if an agreed protocol for the particular condition has been followed. These changes involve direct communication between GPs and consultants of a type which has not taken place before.

These changes have happened at a time when doctors' referral patterns are being analysed in greater detail, and when doctors are also being encouraged to audit the care they offer to their patients. The development of referral guidelines, described in Chapters 11 and 12, has also been catalysed by these changes, and these again involve a new type of communication between GPs and consultants to try to establish which patients will derive greatest benefit from specialist referral.

The changes in the NHS also potentially involve a shift of power away from secondary care to the primary care purchasers (fundholders, or HAs on behalf of non-fundholders), which again may alter quite fundamentally the way that professional groups relate to each other. In the same way that 1948 was a watershed in health service development in the UK, with the formal division of the NHS into primary and secondary care, 1991 is likely to be seen as a time in which fundamental changes in the relationship between GPs and specialists took place.

Conclusion

This chapter shows that there are a number of areas where communication between general practitioners and specialists could be improved. Indeed, it could be argued that communication between doctors is the weakest part of the referral process. The most obvious potential for change lies in improving existing standard forms of written communication between general practitioners and hospital doctors. However, the changing relationship between doctors working in primary and secondary care, and the increased emphasis on definition of minimum standards within the NHS may produce more radical changes in the ways in which doctors communicate. These changes are likely to be to the benefit of doctors' satisfaction with the referral process and to result in improved patient care.

References

Bado, W. and Williams, C.J. (1984). Usefulness of letters from hospitals to general practitioners. *British Medical Journal* **288**, 1813–4.

Beyer, J.M., Horslev-Petersen, K., and Helin, P. (1985). Shuttle case records: link between general practice and the specialist unit. *British Medical Journal* **290**, 677–80.

Blaney, D. and Pullen, I. (1989). Communication between psychiatrists and general practitioners: what style of letters do psychiatrists prefer? *Journal of the Royal College of General Practitioners* **39**, 67.

Brown, R.M.A., Strathdee, G., Christie-Brown, J.R.W., and Robinson, P.H. (1988). A comparison of referrals to primary care and hospital outpatient clinics. *British Journal of Psychiatry* **153**, 168–73.

Browning, S.M., Ford, M.F., Goddard, C.A., and Brown, A.C. (1987). A psychiatric clinic in general practice — a description and comparison with an outpatient clinic. *Bulletin of the Royal College of Psychiatrists* **11**, 114–7.

Claoué, C. and Elkington, A.R. (1986). Informing the hospital of patients' drug regimes. *British Medical Journal* **292**, 101.

Craddock, N. and Craddock, B. (1989). Psychiatric discharge summaries: differing requirements of psychiatrists and general practitioners. *British Medical Journal* **299**, 1382.

Creed, F. and Marks, B. (1989). Liaison psychiatry in general practice: a comparison of the liaison-attachment scheme and shifted outpatient clinic models. *Journal of the Royal College of General Practitioners* **39**, 514–7.

De Alarcon, R. and Hodson, J.M. (1964). Value of the general practitioner's letter — a further study in medical communication. *British Medical Journal* **2**, 435–8.

Doeleman, F. (1987). Improving communication between general practitioners and specialists. *Family Practice* **4**, 176–82.

Dowie, R. (1983). General practitioners and consultants, a study of outpatient referrals. King Edward's Hospital Fund for London, London.

Draper, J., Field, S., Thomas, H., and Hare, M.J. (1986). Should women carry their antenatal records? *British Medical Journal* **292**, 603.

Dunn, D.C. and Dale, R.F. (1986). Combined computer generated discharge documents and surgical audit. *British Medical Journal* **292**, 816–8.

Ezedum, S. and Kerr, D.N.S. (1977). Collaborative care of hypertensives using a shared record. *British Medical Journal* **2**, 1402–3.

Ferguson, B. (1987). Psychiatric clinics in general practice — an asset for primary care. *Health Trends* **19**, 22.

Gilchrist, W.J., Lee, Y.C., Tam, H.C., MacDonald, J.B., and Williams, B.O. (1987). Prospective study of drug reporting by general practitioners for an elderly population referred to a geriatric service. *British Medical Journal* **294**, 289–90.

Grace, J.F., and Armstrong, D. (1987). Reasons for referral to hospital: Extent of agreement between the perceptions of patients, general practitioners and consultants. *Family Practice* **3**, 143–7.

Hall, M.H., McIntyre, S., and Porter, M. (1985). *Antenatal care assessed.* Aberdeen University Press, Aberdeen.

Harding, J. (1987). Study of discharge communications from hospital doctors to an Inner London general practice. *Journal of the Royal College of General Practitioners* **37**, 494–5.

Hartog, M. (1988). Medical outpatients. *Journal of the Royal College of Physicians* **22**, 51.

Health Visitors Association, Royal College of General Practitioners, General Medical Services Committee of the British Medical Association, British Paediatric Association (1990). *Report of the Joint Working Party on Professional and Parent Held Records used in Child Health Surveillance.* British Paediatric Association, London.

Hill, R.D. (1976). Community care services for diabetics in the Poole area. *British Medical Journal* **1**, 1137–9.

Howard, D.J. (1986). Structured discharge letter in a department of geriatric medicine. *Health Trends* **18**, 12–13.

Jacobs, L.G.H and Pringle, M.A. (1990). Referral letters and replies from orthopaedic departments: opportunities missed. *British Medical Journal* **301**, 470–3.

Jones, R.B., Hedley, A.J., Allison, S.P., and Tattershall, R.B. (1988). Censoring of patient held records by doctors. *Journal of the Royal College of General Practitioners* **38**, 117–8.

Juncosa, S., Jones, R.B., and McGhee, S.M. (1990). Appropriateness of hospital referral for hypertension. *British Medical Journal* **300**, 646–8.

Long, A. and Atkins, J.B. (1974). Communications between general practitioners and consultants. *British Medical Journal* **4**, 456–9.

MacFarlane, A. and Saffin, K. (1990). Do general practitioners and health visitors like 'parent held' child health records. *British Journal of General Practice* **40**, 106–8.

Mageean, R.J. (1986). Study of 'discharge communications' from hospital. *British Medical Journal* **293**, 1283–4.

McGlade, K., Bradley, T., Murphy, G.J.J., and Lundy, G.P.P. (1988). Referral to hospital by general practitioners: a study of compliance and communication. *British Medical Journal* **297**, 1246–8.

Mitchell, A.R.K. (1983). Liaison psychiatry in general practice. *British Journal of Hospital Medicine* **30**, 100–6.

Mitchell, A.R.K. (1985). Psychiatrists in primary health care settings. *British Medical Journal* **147**, 371–9.

Morrison, W.G. and Pennycook, A.G. (1991). A study of the content of general practitioners' referral letters to an accident and emergency department. *British Journal of Clinical Practice* **45**, 95–6.

Newton, J., Eccles, M., and Hutchinson, A. (1992). Communication between general practitioners and consultants: what should their letters contain?. *British Medical Journal* **304**, 821–4.

NHS Management Executive (1990). The Care Card — evaluation of the Exmouth Project. Her Majesty's Stationery Office, London.

Penny, T.M. (1988). Delayed communication between hospitals and general practitioners. *British Medical Journal* **297**, 28–9.

Porter, K.M. and Chapple, C. (1985). Hospital discharge letters for orthopaedic patients — what does the general practitioner want? *Health Trends* **17**, 42–4.

Price, D., Cooke, J., Singleton, S., and Feely, M. (1986). Doctors' unawareness of the drugs their patients are taking: a major cause of overprescribing. *British Medical Journal* **292**, 99–100.

Pringle, M. (1989). What benefits do general practitioners see in electronic links to hospitals, family practitioner committees and community services? *Health Trends* **21**, 126–8.

Pullen, I.M. and Yellowlees, A.J. (1985). Is communication improving between general practitioners and psychiatrists. *British Medical Journal* **290**, 31–3.

Roland, M.O., Bewley, B. (1992). BONELINE: evaluation of an initiative to improve telephone communication between general practitioners and specialists. *Journal of Public Health Medicine.* In press.

Sandler, D.A. and Mitchell, J.R.A. (1987). Interim discharge summaries: how are they best delivered to general practitioners. *British Medical Journal* **295**, 1523–5.

Sandler, D.A., Heaton, C., Garner, S.T., and Mitchell, J.R.A. (1989). Patients' and general practitioners' satisfaction with information given on discharge from hospital: audit of a new information card. *British Medical Journal* **299**, 1511–3.

Strathdee, G. and Williams, P. (1984). A survey of psychiatrists in primary care: the silent growth of a new service. *Journal of the Royal College of General Practitioners* **34**, 615–8.

Strathdee, G. (1988). Psychiatrists in primary care: the general practitioner viewpoint. *Family Practice* **5**, 111–5.

Thomas, H., Draper, J., Field, S., and Hare, M.J. (1987). Evaluation of an integrated community antenatal clinic. *Journal of the Royal College of General Practitioners* **37**, 544–7.

Tulloch, A.J., Fowler, G.H., MacMullan, J.J., and Spence, J.M. (1975). Hospital discharge reports: content and design. *British Medical Journal* **2**, 443–5.

Westerman, R.F., Hull, F.M., Bezemer, P.D., and Gort, G. (1990). A study of communication between general practitioners and specialists. *British Journal of General Practice* **40**, 445–9.

Wilkin, D. and Smith, A. (1987). Explaining variation in general practitioner referrals to hospital. *Family Practice* **4**, 160–9.

Williams, P. and Wallace, B.B. (1974). General Practitioners and psychiatrists — do they communicate? *British Medical Journal* **1**, 505–7.

Zander, L.I., Watson, M., Taylor, R.W., and Morrell, D.C. (1978). Integration of general practitioner and specialist antenatal care. *Journal of the Royal College of General Practitioners* **28**, 455–8.

9 The patient's perspective

Angela Coulter

Introduction — A different perspective

The patient's perspective has been relatively neglected in research on referrals. GPs' referral patterns have been studied extensively and a number of small-scale studies have elicited GPs' and hospital consultants' views about referrals, but one has to dig deep into the literature to uncover any references to patients' experiences of the referral process.

One of the few studies that did address the issue of patients' views has provided evidence that patients often have a different perspective on referrals from that of the GP or the specialist involved in their care. Grace and Armstrong (1986, 1987) gave questionnaires to 306 patients referred to hospital outpatient clinics asking for their views on the reason for the referral, whether they thought their GP could have done more before referring them, whether they considered the referral was necessary, and whether they felt they had been referred to the most suitable consultant. The same questions were asked of the GP and the consultant involved.

Grace and Armstrong found that patients and GPs agreed on the reason for the referral in only 49.3 per cent of the cases, and all three parties agreed in only one third. In the light of this disagreement about the purpose of referral, it was not surprising that there was also disagreement about the necessity and suitability of many of the referrals; patient, GP, and specialist were in complete agreement that the referral was necessary in only 29.6 per cent of the referrals studied.

It seems clear, then, that patients have a distinctive perspective on the referral process, which can be distinguished from that of the medical professionals. In order to understand this better we shall consider two key points in the process of being referred to a specialist: the patient's role in the decision to refer, and the patient's experience of the outpatient consultation.

The patient's role in the decision to refer

As we have seen in Chapter 7, the decision about whether or not to refer a patient for specialist attention is often a difficult and complex one. In a situation where a GP is uncertain about the best course of action, he or she may be influenced either directly or indirectly by the views and attitudes of the patient. There are a number of ways in which patients can exert an influence on the GP's decision to refer.

Patient-initiated referrals

Dowie interviewed 64 GPs about their referral behaviour (Dowie 1983). She identified four different ways in which, according to the GPs, referrals could be initiated by patients:

1. The first situation arises when a patient presents with a clinical condition knowing full well that their GP will have to refer them on for specialist attention because of the nature or complexity of their condition. In most cases this referral is straightforward, although some GPs in Dowie's study expressed resentment when patients' demands were too direct, making them feel that they were being used simply as a referral agency.

2. The second situation described by Dowie applies to patients who want prophylactic interventions, notably vasectomy and sterilization, or termination of pregnancy. GPs saw these as legitimate reasons for patient-initiated request, although the decision was shared to the extent that it was discussed in the consultation prior to referral.

3. The third type of patient-initiated referral is also, to some extent, a shared decision. This occurs when a GP has been trying to establish a diagnosis or an effective treatment strategy for some time without success. If the patient or a relative suggests that it might be time to seek specialist advice, the GP may welcome the suggestion as a way out of the dilemma.

4. The fourth type of patient referral initiative is much more problematic for the GP. This is when the patient demands to see a specialist, but the GP considers that there are no clinical grounds for referral. The GP is then caught in a difficult situation: to refer may risk invoking the disapproval of the consultant who could see this referral as a waste of time, but on the other hand the relationship with the patient may be harmed if referral is refused. Some of the GPs in Dowie's study described their attempts to cope with this dilemma by concurring with the demand for referral, but including a hint in the letter to the consultant that it was made at the patient's request.

There is very little documented evidence of the extent to which patients exert direct influence on clinical decision-making in the NHS. Szasz and Hollender (1956) described three basic models of the doctor–patient relationship: activity–passivity, guidance–co-operation, and mutual participation. In the first of these models the patient is an entirely passive recipient of the doctor's actions, as is often the case in severe injuries or other emergency situations. The second model, guidance–co-operation, still underlies much of medical practice. This model describes an imbalance of power between doctor and patient, in which the patient co-operates in whatever action the doctor deems appropriate without argument or disagreement. The model of mutual participation, on the other hand, assumes that both participants in an interaction have approximately equal power. In this case the relationship is a partnership in which the doctor helps the patient to help him or herself. This situation is what most GPs are aiming to achieve in the management of chronic diseases, such as diabetes.

In his discussion of Szasz and Hollender's models, Friedson argued that they were incomplete because they ignored the possibility that the patient could ever assume a dominant role (Friedson 1970). He asserted that this is possible in certain situations and he cited the example of high-status patients in a client-dependent situation, such as private practice, where the doctor is dependent on the patronage of the patient. If patients are sometimes able to exert some control over the decision-making process, we should add another type of relationship to the list of typologies. We shall call this the consumer sovereignty model.

Social class differences in referral patterns

Following Freidson's argument, if we are searching for evidence of patients' influence on referral decision-making in general practice, we might look for social class differences in referral patterns. If the consumer sovereignty model is a reality in general practice, one could plausibly expect to find that patients in the higher social classes or private patients are more likely to be referred, all else being equal, than those in working class groups.

The classic example of an effect of patient demand on clinical decision-making is tonsillectomy. When this operation was at the height of its popularity — around a third of all British children had their tonsils removed in the 1930s and 1940s — tonsillectomy rates were characterized by dramatic social class differences. The children of social class I and II families were much more likely to undergo this operation than were those in social classes IV and V (Coulter and McPherson 1985). It seems most unlikely that the need for this operation was greater among middle class children, so the social class gradient in tonsillectomy rates is usually taken as evidence of the superior ability of middle class parents to obtain what was then seen as a desirable health care intervention. Tonsillectomy is much less fashionable nowadays, but its declining use has been paralleled by an increase in the rate at which another ENT operation, myringotomy, is performed. Interestingly, this operation is also more common among children from higher social classes (Black 1985).

It is hard to know whether these social class differences in elective surgical rates are the result of differential rates of referral by GPs or differences in the way specialists assess patients for surgery. As we have seen in Chapter 6, the evidence on social class differences in referral rates is rather confusing. Some studies have found a social class gradient with higher referral rates for patients in the professional or middle class groups, while others have found the opposite pattern (Wilkin and Smith 1987).

Social influences on the referral decision

It is perhaps not surprising that no clear social class pattern emerges when one examines all referral decisions in aggregate. One would not expect the consumer sovereignty model to apply in the majority of referral decision. Differences are much more likely to emerge where the decision is not clear-cut, or where there is doubt about the most appropriate course of action.

A qualitative or ethnographic approach may be a better way of studying the doctor–patient relationship if one wants to assess the different factors influencing the decision to refer. This was the approach adopted in a study of referrals to two psychiatric outpatient clinics (Morgan 1989). Most of the patients studied had consulted their GP in the first instance for a physical disorder. GPs investigated or treated these in the conventional manner until they suspected that the problem might be 'psychiatric'. The psychiatric referral was usually triggered by persistent consultations for physical symptoms which did not respond to drug therapy or reassurance, often coupled with increasing difficulties in the GP's relationship with the patient.

In 38 per cent of the 106 cases studied, the patient or their relatives requested referral to a specialist when the GP's management of the condition did not appear to be succeeding. In some of these cases the GP acted simply as an administrative agent, arranging clinic appointments in response to direct requests from the patient or their relatives. Sometimes the ulterior motives for these requests were clear; for example, to obtain better council accommodation, improved working conditions, sickness benefits, or the resolution of marital conflicts. Morgan found that the severity of their symptoms was a weak predictor of the circumstances in which patients were referred to psychiatric clinics. In the referrals he studied, the route to specialist care was strongly influenced by social factors as well as clinical events.

GPs' perceptions of patients' pressure

In most cases the issue of whether GPs are subjected to overt pressure from patients to refer them to a specialist has been looked at from the GP's point of view, rather than that of the patient. Armstrong *et al.* (1991) asked 160 GPs to keep records of all the referrals they made during one week. As well as identifying each referral as it occurred, they recorded the reason for the referral, whether it was a private or NHS referral, the specialty of the referral, and their perceptions of the degree of pressure exerted by the patient for the referral. In 61 per cent of the 862 referrals made during the week the GPs reported that there was no pressure from the patient to refer, in 26 per cent the GPs reported a little pressure, and in 13 per cent they felt there was much pressure. Pressure was greater from patients referred privately and from those referred to clinics in psychiatry, rheumatology, dermatology, and orthopaedics. GPs with the highest referral rates were significantly more likely to report pressure from patients.

As the authors of this study were keen to emphasize, patient pressure as measured in this study relates only to the GPs' perceptions. It is possible that in some cases the patient exerted pressure but the GP failed to appreciate it or, conversely, that the patient was not exerting pressure but was perceived as doing so. However, whether the pressure is real or not, it does seem possible that GPs' perceptions of pressure from their patients may explain some of the variation in referral rates.

A study of 450 referrals to an orthopaedic clinic looked at patients, GPs', and consultants views of the referral (Roland *et al.* 1991). This study found similar levels of disagreement between consultants and GPs as to the appropriateness of the referral as was reported in Grace and Armstrong's study (1987). In 10.8 per cent of cases the GP who had made the referral said they thought it was probably or definitely unnecessary. This was more likely to be the case where GPs felt they had been under pressure from the patient. Consultants in this study stated that 43 per cent of the referrals were possibly or definitely inappropriate, in most cases because they felt the GP could have handled the problem. Nevertheless, the majority of patients (82.7 per cent) felt they had been helped by seeing the specialist.

The authors of this study quote the example of a patient referred with a ganglion; the GP reported a lot of pressure to refer, the consultant rated the referral as 'possibly inappropriate' as the patient did not wish to have surgery, but the patient commented that 'It was very helpful and useful. I was very satisfied.' This example highlights the confusion which often exists about the reason for referral. The patient's wish for explanation and reassurance is often not seen as a legitimate reason for referral by consultants and is often not communicated to them by GPs.

Patients' views of the need for second opinions

There have been few studies of patients' views of the need for referral, in particular whether there is a significant demand for referral which is unrecognized or ignored by GPs. One exception was the College of Health survey of a representative sample of 2338 adults in the UK to investigate the extent to which there was an unmet demand for second opinions for medical problems (College of Health 1991). Nearly one in five (436 people) of those surveyed said they had wanted a second opinion in the last two years.

The reasons given for wanting to see another doctor included 31 per cent who said they were not getting any better on their current treatment, 30 per cent wanted the reassurance of another opinion, 29 per cent were not confident that their doctor knew enough about the condition, 20 per cent said they could not get enough information from their doctor, 19 per cent said their doctor could not give them a diagnosis, 17 per cent felt their doctor did not understand properly, 12 per cent did not trust their doctor completely, 11 per cent wanted to be sure the proposed treatment was necessary, and 4 per cent did not like the side-effects of the treatment they had been given.

However, only about a third of those who wanted a second opinion had actually asked for one. Of those who did ask, only 10 per cent were refused. The authors of this report argued that requests for second opinions should not be refused and they suggested that these requests could sometimes be met by referral to other GPs rather than to hospital specialists.

Self-referral

Self-referral to hospital specialists is not normally available to NHS patients, although it sometimes occurs in the private sector. Officially, NHS patients can only refer themselves directly to accident and emergency departments, to genito-urinary clinics, and in exceptional cases to certain other emergency services — for example, open access clinics for children with asthma. In practice, direct access to specialist outpatient clinics bypassing the referral system does sometimes occur, especially among patients who have been frequent outpatient attenders in the past and who have come to know the staff of the outpatient department.

One way in which patients can obtain a second opinion without formal referral by their GP is to refer themselves to non-orthodox practitioners. In 1987, it has been estimated, there were around 1900 qualified, non-medical practitioners of acupuncture, chiropractic, homeopathy, naturopathy, and osteopathy practicing in the UK (Thomas *et al.* 1991). Of the estimated 70 600 patients seen by this group of practitioners in an average week, most (78 per cent) were attending with a musculoskeletal problem. The majority of these patients continued to rely on conventional general practitioner and specialist care for other health problems, and 18 per cent were receiving conventional treatment concurrently for the same problem.

The other main route to specialist care which is open to all patients is self-referral to an accident and emergency department. There has long been concern, particularly in metropolitan areas, that a substantial proportion of patients attending accident and emergency departments have conditions which could be adequately managed by their GP.

In one south London general practice the partners provided 24-hour cover and made themselves available to see urgent cases even when surgeries were fully booked (Singh 1988). Despite this, they estimated that their patients' use of accident and emergency consultations during the course of a year amounted to the equivalent of 70 surgeries. Most accident and emergency attendances occurred during the hours when the general practice surgery was open. On being asked why they had bypassed their GP and gone direct to the accident and emergency department, 41 per cent of the patients said it was because their problem was urgent, 24 per cent said they thought they would need an X-ray, 18 per cent said they thought their doctor would not be available, and 7 per cent thought that they would be seen more quickly in casualty.

Cartwright and Anderson (1981) reported similar comments by patients who had attended casualty departments. Some of their respondents indicated that they had more confidence in the ability of hospital staff to deal with their problem. Others said they went directly to the hospital because they did not want to waste their GP's time.

Rising expectations

There is some evidence that patients' expectations of the benefits and availability of specialist care are rising. Cartwright and Anderson reported an increasing trend in the proportion of patients who expected to be referred to hospital for injuries or minor surgical procedures. In their 1964 study 12 per cent of respondents said they would expect to be referred for a sprained ankle, whereas by 1977 the proportion had risen to 23 per cent; the proportion expecting referral for removal of a small cyst rose from 37 per cent in 1964 to 51 per cent in 1977; 20 per cent expected referral for treatment of an abscess in 1964, rising to 34 per cent in 1977. However, the majority of patients in their studies (79 per cent in 1964 and 71 per cent in 1977) expressed a preference for a health service centred, as at present, on GP consultation with referral when necessary, rather than one in which there would be free access to specialists.

The studies described above provide evidence of a considerable demand from patients for access to specialist advice, as a supplement rather than a substitute for normal GP care. Often the reassurance of a second opinion is all that is required. This demand may not always be accepted as legitimate by medical practitioners. In particular, specialists often assume that patients have been referred to their clinics so that the specialists can take over the management of the problem. This can result in unnecessary duplication of effort and numerous repeat appointments in the outpatients clinic for conditions which could be equally well or better managed in general practice. Failure to understand and communicate the patient's views and needs can result in conflict between the GP and the specialist. If the specialist misunderstands the factors prompting the decision to refer, the GP may be blamed for referring unnecessarily.

The patient's experience of the outpatient consultation

Most studies of patients' experiences of attending outpatient clinics have focused on organizational issues. Many of these have been initiated by hospital managers concerned to establish the views of users with a view to making improvements in the services they run. Since more people attend outpatient clinics than any other hospital service — there were approximately 40 million outpatient attendances in England and Wales in 1988/9 — it is encouraging that there is an increasing focus on this aspect of patient care. There are considerable difficulties in the design and interpretation of patient satisfaction research (Locker and Dunt 1978; Fitzpatrick 1984), but systematic measurement of the experience of attending outpatient departments is being actively encouraged, so it is likely that such studies will proliferate (McIver 1991).

The issues on which patients have been found to have pronounced views include the following: ease of access to the hospital or clinic, convenience of appointment times, travel and parking arrangements, signposting, and so on; waiting times between referral and appointment, and time spent waiting in the clinic; the waiting environment and facilities; and communication between staff and patients, including the provision of written material.

One of the most comprehensive surveys of patients' experiences of outpatients departments was carried out for the Royal Commission on the National Health Service in 1977/8 (Royal Commission 1978). The researchers interviewed 2267 patients who had attended outpatient clinics throughout the UK. Many other surveys have been carried out in outpatients clinics since this one and the major concern in the majority of these has been waiting-times in the clinics (Dixon and Carr-Hill 1989).

Waiting for the appointment

Over half of the patients in the Royal Commission survey had received an outpatient appointment within three weeks of the referral letter. A substantial proportion of those who were kept waiting longer than this said they were upset by the wait, either because they were concerned to know what was wrong with them, or because they were suffering physical pain or discomfort. Some patients were worried that the hospital had forgotten about them because they had not been sent an appointment date. Waiting-times for outpatient appointments are now much longer than three weeks in many areas and this continues to be a cause for concern to many patients and their GPs (see Chapter 11).

Long waiting-times for appointment are obviously an important source of dissatisfaction for patients, but they are also both a result and a cause of inefficient organization. Two recent studies have found a relationship between appointment dates and non-attendance rates. McGlade *et al.*

(1988) studied non-attendance rates among patients referred to outpatient clinics from their west Belfast practice Fifteen per cent of the 269 patients they had referred failed to attend the appointment. Significantly more of the patients who had to wait more than two months for an appointment failed to attend than those whose appointment was within two months of referral. Frankel and colleagues (1989) warn against blaming the patients for non-attendance. In their case-control study of attenders and non-attenders they found few differences in the severity of the clinical condition for which they were referred, but the non-attenders were more likely to experience practical difficulties in getting to the hospital, and they were much more likely than attenders to have received very short notice of their appointments; 50 per cent received one week's notice or less. The most commonly reported reasons for non-attendance were being on holiday (28 per cent), thinking treatment unnecessary (12 per cent), difficulties getting off work (12 per cent), the hospital altering the appointment (9 per cent), and feeling too unwell on the day (9 per cent).

Getting to the hospital

It may not always be evident to those initiating outpatient appointments that some patients experience considerable difficulties in making arrangements to travel to the hospital. Patients with their own cars face difficulties if the hospital has inadequate parking space, those who depend on public transport can be affected by the cost or inconvenience of the service, and those for whom hospital transport is provided sometimes have to suffer a long wait for collection or return delivery. However, the Royal Commission survey found little evidence of unmet demand for hospital transport, which is mainly used by elderly patients; only 5 per cent of those who made their own way to hospital said they would have preferred the hospital to have laid on transport (Royal Commission 1978).

The imposition of car parking charges and the increasingly stringent measures being adopted by hospital managements to deter parking in restricted areas — for example, wheel clamps — place an additional burden on patients attending hospital clinics. One fundholding practice discovered to its surprise that many patients opted for referral to a district general hospital in preference to the three teaching hospitals with which the practice had contracts, simply because parking arrangements were more convenient (Laurance 1991).

Waiting in the clinic

Once in the outpatient department, the Royal Commission researchers found that most patients were reasonably satisfied with the facilities in the waiting room, although some felt that more toys should be provided for children. However, there was a certain amount of dissatisfaction about the length of time spent waiting to see the doctor; 28 per cent of those who had to wait more than 15 minutes felt that the waiting-time was unreasonable and, not surprisingly, the proportion who were dissatisfied increased with the length of the wait. The majority of patients said they would prefer to be given a specific appointment time, although a few patients said that open appointment times suited their domestic arrangements better.

Communication

A common feature of studies of patient satisfaction is the finding that many patients would like more information about their condition and its treatment. Twenty five per cent of the outpatients in the Royal Commission survey said they would have liked more information about how they were getting on, but a large proportion of these said they felt unable to ask the doctors for this information. The main reason given for this reluctance to ask the doctors to tell them what they wanted to know was that patients found their manner abrupt and off-putting. Others said that the doctors seemed in too much of a hurry or too busy to deal with their questions. Fifteen per cent of outpatients reported difficulties in understanding what they were told. Sometimes this was due to failure to understand medical terminology, and sometimes due to the doctors' lack of clarity in expression. Doctors appeared to take more care to explain examinations and treatment in everyday language to elderly patients than to younger ones; it was the latter who reported more difficulties in comprehension.

Effective communication and an ability to understand the patient's perspective may be important in promoting healing. Two studies of patients referred to outpatient clinics for common problems — headaches and back pain — have suggested that satisfaction with the outpatient consultation might be related to clinical outcome.

Fitzpatrick and colleagues (1983) interviewed 95 patients who had been referred to neurology outpatient clinics for headaches. The patients were interviewed prior to their first hospital consultation and again between two and three weeks afterwards. One year later 75 of the sample were re-interviewed. The patients concerns at the initial interview fell into three groups; one group expressed worries that their symptoms might be due to a serious disorder such as a brain tumour, another group wanted expert and up-to-date advice on symptom relief, and the third group hoped for advice on the underlying causes of their symptoms and ways in which they could modify their lifestyle to prevent recurrence. At the second interview, which was conducted soon after the outpatient visit and before any change in symptoms had been noted, patients' satisfaction with the consultation varied markedly. Thirty six per cent were dissatisfied, either with the medical actions initiated by the doctor, or with the communication and explanations provided, or for both reasons. The most dissatisfied group was those who had hoped for detailed discussion of lifestyle factors which might be responsible for causing or exacerbating their symptoms. By the time of the third interview symptoms had improved for over half of the sample. Those who had been satisfied with the outpatient consultation were significantly more likely to report improvement than those who were not.

A before-and-after design was also used for the second study, of patients referred by their GPs to a rheumatological back pain clinic (Fitzpatrick *et al*. 1987). 72 patients were interviewed at home before their outpatient appointment and 69 per cent of these completed a postal questionnaire three months after the first clinic visit. Prior to the outpatient appointment the actions most frequently expected by patients were: learning from the clinic how to avoid pressures and strains on the back (94 per cent), having the doctor explain the reasons for any tests or investigations which might be necessary (94 per cent), and having an opportunity to discuss the future prospects of the back problem with the doctor (89 per cent). Patients were much less likely to say that they expected to receive treatment; only 34 per cent said they expected to be prescribed medication for back pain, 28 per cent thought they would be considered for surgery, and 19 per cent expected acupuncture. Two-thirds of the patients were satisfied with the outpatient consultation, but the remainder were dissatisfied with the information they were given about the future prospects of their back pain, or the doctor's failure to encourage discussion of their personal worries. The satisfaction rating was positively correlated with improvements in pain and disability scores at the post-appointment assessment.

Neither of these studies should be taken as conclusive evidence of a positive effect of good communication style on clinical outcomes. There are considerable methodological problems in establishing such a relationship and there are many other plausible explanations for these findings. However, they do underscore the value of eliciting patients' concerns and expectations so that these can be addressed (Pendleton *et al*. 1984). The studies demonstrate that patients often have a realistic view of the likely effectiveness of treatment, but would like more information about the nature of their problem and its prognosis than is often provided.

Conclusion

The evidence outlined in this chapter points to the need for greater understanding of the patient's perspective. This is important both in assessing the appropriateness of referral decisions and in evaluating the outcomes of referral. The role of specialist referral in providing advice and reassurance, as well as diagnosis and treatment, is important to patients and should not therefore be undervalued by doctors.

References

Armstrong, D., Fry, J., and Armstrong, P. (1991). Doctors' perceptions of pressure from patients for referral. *British Medical Journal* **302**, 1186–8.

Black, N. (1985). Glue ear: the new dyslexia? *British Medical Journal* **290**, 1963–5.

Cartwright, A. and Anderson, R. (1981). *General practice revisited.* Tavistock, London.

College of Health (1991). *Which? way to health.* February, 32–5.

Coulter, A., McPherson, K. (1985) Socioeconomic variations in the use of common surgical operations. *British Medical Journal* **291**, 183–7.

Dixon, P. and Carr-Hill, R. (1989) *The NHS and its customers: Booklet 3 — Customer feedback surveys: a review of current practice.* Centre for Health Economics, University of York.

Dowie, R. (1983). *General practitioners and consultants: a study of outpatient referrals.* King Edward's Hospital Fund for London, London.

Fitzpatrick, R. (1984). Satisfaction with health care. *In* R. Fitzpatrick, J. Hinton, S. Newman, G. Scambler, J. Thompson (ed.) *The experience of illness* Tavistock, London.

Fitzpatrick, R., Hopkins, A., and Harvard-Watts, O. (1983). Social dimensions of healing: a longitudinal study of outcomes of medical management of headaches *Social Science and Medicine* **17**, 501–10.

Fitzpatrick, R., Bury, M., Frank, A., and Donnelly, T. (1987). Problems in the assessment of outcome in a back pain clinic. *International Journal of Disability Studies* **9**, 161–5.

Frankel, S., Farrow, A., and West, R. (1989). Non-attendance or non-invitation? A case-control study of failed outpatient appointments. *British Medical Journal* **298**, 1343–5.

Freidson, E. (1970). *The profession of medicine.* Dodd Mead & Co, New York.

Grace, J.F. and Armstrong, D. (1986). Reasons for referral to hospital: extent of agreement between the perceptions of patients, general practitioners and consultants. *Family Practice* **3**, 143–7.

Grace, J.F. and Armstrong, D. (1987). Referral to hospital: perceptions of patients, general practitioners and consultants about necessity and suitability of referral *Family Practice* **4**, 170–5.

Laurance, J. (1991). The Freeman Hospital *British Medical Journal* **303**, 765–6.

Locker, D. and Dunt, D. (1978). Theoretical and methodological issues in socio-logical studies of consumer satisfaction with medical care. *Social Science and Medicine* **12**, 283–92.

McGlade, K., Bradley, T., Murphy, G., and Lundy, G. (1988). Referrals to hospital by general practitioners: a study of compliance and communication *British Medical Journal* **297**, 1246–8.

McIver, S. (1991). *Obtaining the views of outpatients.* King's Fund Centre, London.

Morgan, D. (1989). Psychiatric cases: an ethnography of the referral process. *Psychological Medicine* **19**, 743–53.

Pendleton, D., Schofield, T., Tate, P., and Havelock, P. (1984). *The consultation: an approach to learning and teaching.* Oxford University Press, Oxford.

Roland, M.O., Porter, R.W., Matthews, J.G., Redden, J.F., Simonds, G.W. and Bewley, B. (1991). Improving care: a study of orthopaedic outpatient referrals *British Medical Journal* **302**, 1124–8.

Royal Commission on the National Health Service (1978). *Patients' attitudes to the hospital service.* Her Majesty's Stationery Office, London.

Singh, S. (1988). Self referral to accident and emergency department: patients' perceptions. *British Medical Journal* **297**, 1179–80.

Szasz, T.S. and Hollender, M.H. (1956). A contribution to the philosophy of medicine. *Archives of Internal Medicine* **97**, 585–92.

Thomas, K.J., Carr, J., Westlake, L., and Williams, B.T. (1991). Use of non-orthodox and conventional health care in Great Britain. *British Medical Journal* **302**, 207–10.

Wilkin, D. and Smith, A. (1987). Explaining variation in general practitioner referrals to hospital. *Family Practice* **4**, 160–9.

10 Measuring appropriateness of hospital referrals

Martin Roland

Introduction — Why measure appropriateness?

A child living in the Soke of Peterborough is nineteen times more likely to undergo tonsillectomy than one living in Cambridgeshire . . . it is difficult to believe that all subjects for operation are selected with true discrimination.

This quotation from Glover's paper (Glover 1938) over 50 years ago is a reminder that variations in medical practice and appropriateness of treatment are not new subjects for study. Before discussing appropriateness of hospital referrals in detail, it is important to understand what is meant by appropriateness.

The first point to appreciate about hospital referral is that the patient, the GP, and the specialist may have different perspectives on what constitutes an appropriate referral. In discussions within the medical literature the patient's judgement is often regarded as subordinate to that of his or her doctors; this balance may need to change if government wishes the health service to become more responsive to the perceived needs of its consumers. A second point about the appropriateness of a referral is that it needs to relate to the reason for that referral. Failure to communicate about the reasons for referral is one reason why specialists and GPs may disagree about the appropriateness of a referral. A third axis to consider in relation to referral is that there is a distinction between medical decisions about appropriate referral (for example, should all patients with rectal bleeding be referred to hospital?) and societal decisions which reflect a wider decision about whether society can afford to or is prepared to pay for certain types of treatment (for example, *in vitro* fertilization, cosmetic surgery). These three dimensions show that a referral cannot simply be judged 'appropriate' or 'inappropriate'; the context in which the referral took place and the standpoint of the judge are important to consider if one is to avoid over-simplistic statements about what treatment is or is not appropriate.

There are a number of reasons why the issue of appropriateness of care has recently been brought into focus. The first relates to the limited volume of health care that can be provided within the NHS. The NHS has always been cash limited — it has had a budget voted for it annually by Parliament — and there has always been rationing. The principal mechanism for rationing hospital care has been waiting-lists, both for inpatient and outpatient treatment, though the mechanism was not usually referred to as rationing. With the 1991 reform of the NHS, rationing became explicit. HAs became purchasers of health care on behalf of their resident populations, and they became distinct from the hospitals, who were the providers. HAs had fixed budgets with which to purchase secondary health care for their patients, and were faced with decisions about what to spend their money on. In order to make best use of resources it became necessary to try and ensure that hospital resources were directed mainly towards those patients who could benefit from them. Optimization of use of hospital resources required, so far as possible, that referrals should be appropriate.

The second reason for an increase in interest in appropriateness of referrals was the increasing documentation of wide variations in referral rates among GPs. This was from an accumulation of research data, reviewed in Chapter 6, which shows persistent and unexplained variation in the number of patients that individual GPs refer to hospital. The existence of variability is not confined to GPs nor to the UK, and there are many other examples of variation in utilization of medical care; for example, admission rates in the UK (Sanders *et al.* 1989) and in the USA (Chassin *et al.* 1986; Wennberg *et al.* 1987; Perrin *et al.* 1989). The phenomenon of variability in medical practice, including referral rates, is not itself evidence of unsatisfactory medical practice although unexplained variation does indicate that there is disagreement between doctors about the management of clinical problems.

There are a number of studies which suggest that there is no clear link between referral rates and the quality or appropriateness of referrals. For example, Knottnerus *et al.* (1990) used an independent expert panel to judge the quality of referrals, and found that high-referring doctors were just as likely to refer appropriately compared to doctors with average referral rates. In a study of referral patterns in the Oxford region, Coulter *et al.* (1990) found that the patients of high-referring doctors were as likely to be admitted to hospital for operations for a number of surgical specialities compared to the patients of low-referring doctors. If the probability that the specialist will arrange hospital admission for a patient following referral can be taken as a marker of the appropriateness of a referral, Coulter's results suggest that the patients of high-referring doctors were no less appropriately referred than the patients of low-referring doctors. In another study Reynolds *et al.* (1991) reported on one practice where doctors with particular areas of expertise appeared to have high rates of referral to those specialties, casting further doubt on the idea that doctors with high referral rates are less competent than those who refer few patients to hospital.

Although one might accept that there is no clear relationship between variation in referral rates and quality of care, variation does nevertheless require explanation. It is likely, though by no means proven, that the costs to the NHS of a low-referring doctor are less than those of a high-referrer; the Government, not surprisingly, would prefer to fund a low spender compared to a high spender unless the latter can demonstrate increased need for medical care or improved patient outcome. Looked at from this angle, the responsibility for demonstrating appropriateness of care shifts firmly to the profession. In order to justify using resources, doctors increasingly will need to demonstrate that they are making appropriate use of resources. This is a major shift in thinking, summarized neatly by Eddy (1990):

What is going on? What is going on is that one of the basic assumptions under-lying the practice of medicine is being challenged. This concerns the intellec-tual foundation of medical care. Simply put, the assumption is that whatever a physician decides is, by definition, correct. The challenge says that while many decisions no doubt are correct, many are not, and elaborate mechanisms are needed to determine which are which.

Interpreting current literature on the appropriateness of hospital referrals

There are a number of papers, usually written by hospital doctors, commenting on the appropriateness of referrals from GPs. By and large these are critical of GPs' referral behaviour. As an example, Sladden and Graham Brown (1989) thought that 26 per cent of their dermatology referrals were unnecessary, and hospital consultants in a range of specialties thought that the GP might have managed without referral in 55 per cent of cases (Grace and Armstrong 1987). The specialties in which referrals are most frequently criticized are rheumatology and orthopaedics (Samantha and Roy 1988; Helliwell and Wright 1991).

In some papers criticism about GPs is extreme; for example, Vigiser *et al.* (1984) found that only 29 per cent of GPs' emergency psychiatric referrals to an Israeli hospital were justified. In other papers, the solution seems extreme; Springall and Todd (1988) used the inaccuracy of dia-gnosis in patients referred with colorectal disease to argue that patients with colorectal symptoms should present directly to hospital.

The results of some papers strongly suggest appropriate referral patterns. As an example, if patients referred for urgent assessment at hospital are admitted to hospital then this suggests that the GP and the admitting physician are in agreement that, for one reason or another, the patient cannot be managed at home. So, for example, Moss *et al.* (1984) found that 91 per cent of 298 patients referred urgently to a general surgical unit in Edinburgh were admitted to hospital, as were 89 per cent of 1500 referrals to an emergency admissions unit in Cambridge (N.T.A. Oswald, personal communication). Indeed, these figures are so high that one might question whether GPs' threshold for requesting assessment for admission is set too high.

There are major problems in the interpretation of this type of paper. The first is that there is likely to have been substantial publication bias in papers reaching publication. It is likely that research into appropriateness of referrals is selectively carried out in specialties or geographical areas where the specialist perceives there to be problems. The author's own work is a good example of this (Roland *et al.* 1991); in a study of 499 orthopaedic referrals to a Doncaster hospital, 213 (43 per cent) were judged to be possibly or definitely inappropriate. However, this setting was chosen for the study precisely because the specialists had complained about their referrals, and a major aim of the study was to identify ways of improving specialists' and GPs' satisfaction with the referral process. It seems highly likely therefore that the results of published work on appropriateness of referral are not generalizable. Further evidence for this comes from a study of specialists' perception of the appropriateness of 600 referrals to six specialties in Cambridge (Fertig and Roland, unpublished data). 20 per cent of 200 referrals to orthopaedics and rheumatology were considered possibly inappropriate, compared to only 4 per cent of 400 referrals to ENT, gynaecology, chest medicine, and ophthalmology. This finding, taken along with the disproportionate number of papers on the appropriateness of referrals for musculo–skeletal problems, suggests that there may be problems in this particular subject area which are again not generalizable. Care should therefore be taken in extrapolating the results of published work on appropriateness beyond the specialties or the geographical areas where the work was carried out.

The second major problem in interpreting the literature on appropriateness of referral is that almost all the studies mentioned (with the exception of Grace and Armstrong 1988) rely on the specialist's own subjective impression of whether or not a referral was appropriate. It is clear from Grace and Armstrong's work that the perceptions of the specialist, the GP, and the patient about the necessity for a referral may be very different. Without any reference to an explicit standard of what constitutes an appropriate referral, it is very difficult to use information on referral patterns to influence behaviour in any kind of rational way. The question of how appropriateness should be measured is therefore central to further discussion on use of hospital sevices.

How should appropriateness be measured?

A number of approaches have been used to measure the appropriateness of referrals. They are in essence no different from methods used to assess the appropriateness of medical care generally, but where data exists they will be illustrated with examples concerning hospital referrals. The four approaches involve:

(1) identification of outliers;

(2) conformity with a protocol;

(3) assessment of outcome;

(4) retrospective identification of missed opportunities.

Identification of outliers

Outliers are those doctors who lie at the extreme ends of a distribution. They deviate from the norm, and in relation to hospital referral include doctors who refer unusually large or small numbers of patients to hospital. When presented with wide variation in referral rates, many commentators have found it irresistible to assume that the 'problem' lay with the outliers. Furthermore, those with responsibility for funding health care will always tend to regard a high-spending outlier as more of a problem than a low-spending outlier. This process has become explicit for prescribing behaviour where high-prescribing GPs in the UK have for many years been visited by government medical officers, with no such attention being given to low-prescribers. Despite the lack of evidence for a relationship between referral rates and quality of referral, conformity to the norm carries with it a persuasive comfortableness, which has been the basis for a number of studies of hospital referrals.

The first group of these are two studies of referrals for abdominal ultrasound (Colquhoun *et al.* 1988; Mills *et al.* 1989). In both studies, a positive pick up rate of 25–30 per cent was found. This was taken as evidence of the value of GP access to X-ray departments, particularly bearing in mind that the results of radiological tests may help GPs to make fewer or more appropriate outpatient referrals (Barton *et al.* 1987). However, the authors of both ultrasound studies used as further evidence of the appropriateness of GP referrals the finding that the positive pick up rate for these examinations was similar to that for referrals from hospital doctors. A similar argument was advanced in relation to endoscopy referrals by Kerrigan *et al.* (1990) who found a similar abnormality rate in referrals from GPs and hospital doctors. This argument is a much weaker one without evidence of appropriate referral by hospital doctors. However, the comfortable assumption is that, if both groups appear to be operating in the same way, they are probably doing the right thing.

The weakness of this argument is well summarized by Mooney and Andersen (1990):

The philosophy of 'cosiness' — all getting together around some common mean or standard and not being an antisocial outlier — can only be seen as virtuous if the point on the scale around which cosiness occurs has some rationale. The challenge here is not variation per se: it is trying to discover where cosiness should occur, and the extent to which it is a virtue.

Conformity to a numeric norm is therefore not a sufficient basis for deciding about appropriateness of referrals. Some direct assessment of quality is necessary.

Conforming with a protocol or guideline

The second method of assessing appropriateness is to develop a protocol or guideline of good clinical practice, and to compare the action of the doctor with that of the protocol. This is a major advance on the subjective opinions of individual specialists in references cited earlier in this chapter. The development of guidelines is regarded by some as a threat to clinical autonomy. The extent to which this is true will depend on the way in which it was generated, and the way in which it is applied. If the guideline is devised as an educational tool for the doctor to use, it poses no threat to autonomy. If, however, payment for a procedure or acceptance of a referral depends on guidelines having been followed, then clinical freedom is restricted. The extent to which this matters depends on whether the guideline can be constructed so that it represents a genuine consensus of relevant opinion based on good evidence. Doctors might reasonably argue that their clinical freedom should not be constrained except by guidelines which meet those conditions. These anxieties aside, the development of guidelines is becoming an important part of the measurement of quality of care in this country, and Chapters 12 and 13 of this book specifically discuss the development and evaluation of referral guidelines. Later in this chapter two particular issues related to guideline development are discussed, namely who should decide what is appropriate, and how disagreement among professionals about what is appropriate practice can be handled.

Assessment of outcome

The third method of measuring the appropriateness of referrals is to measure the outcome of the referral. As an example, Coulter *et al.* (1991) looked at the outcome of a series of gynaecology referrals in terms of the number of referrals which were followed by investigation or operation by the specialist, consultation rates for gynaecological symptoms after the referral, and symptom prevalence following the referral. This approach has the great advantage that some outcome data may be routinely available or readily collected; for example, operation rates, consultation rates. However, there are a number of potential problems with the approach. Firstly, although it may be assumed that certain outcomes indicate that the referral was appropriate — for example, the patient was admitted for operation — this may not be the case. Coulter *et al.* (1990) and Ross *et al.* (1983) have previously shown that the patients of high-referring GPs are as likely to be operated on compared to the patients of low-referring practitioners. This has been adduced as evidence that the patients from the high-referrers are referred just as appropriately as those from low-referrers. An alternative explanation is that the hospital doctors in these studies are indiscriminate in admitting patients for operation, and have a fixed probability of operating when presented with a particular symptom. This issue may be resolved by referral to a guideline for the operation in question to attempt to see whether all the operations done were appropriate.

Looking at symptom prevalence and consultation patterns following referral is in some ways the most attractive outcome measure, since it measures what the doctor really wants for his patient — did the patient get better? However, this outcome measure also needs to be interpreted with some caution. Symptom prevalence would, for example, be an inappropriate outcome measure for referral for back pain, where the natural history is for recovery, unless there were a comparable unreferred group.

Despite these drawbacks, measurement of outcome is likely to become an increasingly important part of medical care evaluation (Ellwood 1988). The Medical Outcomes Study (Tarlov *et al.* 1989) sets out an ambitious programme of outcome measurement in terms of clinical endpoints, physical and social functioning, and patients' health status and satisfaction. These measures are now being applied to a large population. For the great majority of conditions for which GPs refer patients the benefit of referral has not been established in controlled trials, and is unlikely to be. Experience and research over the next few years will determine the extent to which outcome data relating to referral can be used to judge the appropriateness of care.

Retrospective identification of missed opportunities

This method depends on identifying patients with unfavourable health outcomes and looking for ways in which their care could have been improved. Thus, for example, the South Bedfordshire Practitioners' Group (1990) identified missed opportunities for intervention in half of a sample of children with established renal scars, and a number of researchers have analysed the various stages at which delay may occur in the diagnosis of cancer (MacArthur and Smith 1983; Scully *et al.* 1986; Stower 1988). In relation to hospital referral this method is particularly important in that it looks specifically for problems with delay in referral or failure to refer which may be as great a problem as over-referral in terms of optimizing use of health care resources.

Who should measure appropriateness?

If a standard or guideline is used or offered for use by those other than its originators then it is essential that it should be clearly stated who has been involved in making the guideline. As an example, Juncosa *et al.* (1990) described the extent to which referrals for hypertension met two standards. The only description of the development of the standards is that they were 'devised based on published medical opinion'. Since none of the three authors were medically qualified, the standards lacked both expert medical backing and any sense of ownership or validation by the group of doctors to whose referrals they were being applied.

There are three distinct approaches which have been adopted to deciding on standards of appropriate medical care. These are the expert group, the multi-disciplinary consensus group, and the use of a lay panel of judges. These have been used with or without a so called 'Delphi process' of involving a wider group of clinicians.

The expert group

In this approach a panel of experts is assembled in order to decide upon appropriate standards of care for a particular problem. The rationale behind this approach is that the expert in a particular subject is best placed to advise the non-expert on how to deal with a particular problem. This model, which sits easily with the clear pattern of referral from primary to secondary care in the NHS, has a number of drawbacks. The first is that the experts may not agree among themselves, and groups may vary considerably in the extent to which they are supported by analysis of evidence from published literature. Secondly, experts may be regarded as producing standards which cannot be applied in the daily work of the generalist, either because the type of patient that the two doctors see is different, or because the experts have produced a standard which is too rigorous to be applied to the number of patients seen by the generalist, or because the specialist calls for facilities which are not available to the generalist. A third problem is that a standard or guideline is much more likely to be accepted if there is a sense of ownership by the group to whom it is being applied. There is now increasing awareness that decisions about the appropriateness of medical actions need to involve all the parties who are actually making those decisions on a day to day basis.

The multidisciplinary consensus group.

For the reasons described in the previous section, this has become the commonest method for deciding on guidelines for appropriate clinical behaviour. Thus, for example, the authors of a Royal College of Physicians guideline on the management of urinary infection in childhood included five paediatric nephrologists, two paediatricians, two paediatric surgeons, three radiologists, two microbiologists, two GPs, one parent, and a medical co-ordinator (Royal College of Physicians Working Party 1991). Even though the balance of this group is heavily towards specialists, it does contain representation from all the interested professional groups. The approach of using multidisciplinary groups to decide on appropriateness is increasingly becoming the standard, and is used by a number of American health care providers who have been in the forefront of clinical guideline development — for example, RAND Corporation (Brook 1990), and Harvard Community Health Plan (Gottlieb *et al.* 1990).

In relation to referral guidelines, there is an additional reason for involving both GPs and specialists in the development of guidelines which is perhaps more important than the reasons so far mentioned. This relates to the changing nature of the relationship between GPs and specialists. The arrival of the internal market in the NHS and the development of feedback of data to GP on their referral patterns is making it increasingly clear that there are conflicts between complete freedom to refer and efficient operation of the NHS. While covert or overt restriction on referral is an anathema to many, there is no doubt that NHS resources are likely to be more readily available to those who are able to justify their use. There is therefore incentive for specialists and GPs to agree on which patients should be referred, and this is one of the motivations behind the increasing number of specialist/generalist groups developing referral guidelines, which are discussed in more detail in Chapter 12.

Non expert judges

An alternative approach to deciding on appropriateness of medical procedures has been adopted by the King's Fund. In these a panel of judges includes both clinicians and laymen, all of whom are experienced in evaluating evidence, but the judges specifically exclude specialists in the field under consideration. Experts are then invited to present evidence to the judges, in a semi-public forum, and the judges develop their guideline based on their assessment of the evidence presented. This is an interesting approach, and it may become increasingly relevant in a rationed health care system to involve lay people in decisions about what constitutes appropriate medical care. At a recent conference on guideline development, there was strong support for the chairman at least of a guideline development panel not being an expert on the subject in question (Smith 1991).

Delphi process

A feature of a number of approaches to setting standards of appropriate medical care is the Delphi process. This normally involves circulation of a draft guideline for written comments which are then summarized by the person co-ordinating the development of a particular guideline. The circulation may be after an initial literature review, or may follow initial attempts at drafting a guideline by a consensus group. The Delphi process may involve only those people in the group which is developing the guideline, in which case it is used to reduce the number of meetings needed to develop the guideline. Alternatively, circulation is to a wider group to provide input into the guideline from people outside the main development group. Thus, for example, when developing referral guidelines in Cambridge, the medical co-ordinator initially met with one or two consultants in a specialty and with two or three GP trainers. A draft guideline was developed and circulated among the wider group of trainers for comment prior to further refinement.

The Delphi process is an interesting name for this procedure. Certainly the oracle at Delphi was an important source of wisdom in the ancient world. However, one of the characteristics of her advice was its ambiguity. As an example, Socrates, commenting on the Delphic predictions, wrote 'What does the god mean? Why does he not use plain language? . . . This Oracle is his way of telling us that human wisdom has little or no value' (Tredennick 1955). Although it is to be hoped that the modern Delphi process will not gain such a reputation the problem is not without relevance, because one of the features of consensus development of guideline is that it is difficult to get doctors to agree about the appropriateness of clinical procedures.

Consensus pitfalls

These methods of developing clinical guidelines are attractive in that they all produce an agreed form of management that may then be adopted more generally. There are, however, a number of potential pitfalls to this approach.

The first problem is that the extent of literature review prior to guideline writing may be very variable. Few organizations have the resources of the large American agencies which have carried out exhaustive literature reviews prior to the development of guidelines (described in more detail in Chapter 12). It follows that guidelines may ignore or fail to take account of evidence about the effectiveness of particular types of treatment.

Secondly, good evidence may be valued differently under different circumstances. As an example, in terms of actual advice to clinicians, the investigation of patients with transient ischaemic attack may depend largely on the availability of investigative facilities even though there is good evidence that patient benefit would follow investigation.

Thirdly, the content of a guideline may well depend on the composition of the group collected to produce it. As Skrabanek (1990) points out:

The careful selection of participants guarantees a consensus. A token dissident, co-opted to maintain the semblance of impartiality, is, as a rule, not given space to ruffle the smoothness of the consensus report. Yet the very need for consensus stems from a lack of consensus. Why make an issue of agreeing on something that everyone (or nearly everyone) takes for granted.

Can doctors agree about what is appropriate?

Recent attempts to develop consensus guidelines on the appropriateness of medical procedures have highlighted the difficulty in getting doctors to agree about what action is appropriate in a given clinical situation. Quite apart from different interpretations of a clinical situation which relate to observer variability (Feinstein 1985), doctors may differ markedly in their management of the same clinical scenario. As an example, in the UK–TIA aspirin trial, between 0–25 per cent of patients with transient ischaemic attacks had carotid surgery, depending largely on the policy of the neurologist (UK–TIA Study Group 1983). The variation in clinical practice between doctors may relate to their belief in the likely outcome of clinical situations; Eddy (1990) describes the wide variation in the beliefs of specialists about the probability of different outcomes. In addition to divergence of opinion within one health care system, there are of course differences in the way in which doctors in different health care systems will regard appropriateness, given the same data and literature evidence on which to base their opinions (Brook *et al.* 1988; Hopkins *et al.* 1989).

The approach of the RAND corporation to this is to make agreement and disagreement explicit in the guideline development process (Brook 1990). Following detailed literature review and discussion, nine doctors constitute a panel to decide on the clinical appropriateness of a procedure (for example, carotid endarterectomy) for a large number of clinical scenarios. Appropriateness is rated on a scale from 1 (inappropriate) to 9 (appropriate). The procedure is judged appropriate when the median panel rating is 7–9 without disagreement, inappropriate when the median rating is 1–3 and equivocal when it is 4–6. Disagreement is defined as occurring when at least three panel members rate the procedure 1–3 and at least three rate it 7–9. Using this and similar definitions of disagreement, this group have reported that the panel could not agree on appropriate management of between 11 and 29 per cent of a range of medical and surgical conditions (Park *et al.* 1986; Merrick *et al.* 1987).

Conclusion

It is hardly surprising that close scrutiny of medical care should produce areas of disagreement about what treatments are appropriate since so many routine medical procedures have never been evaluated. It is, however, very important that clinical situations where the indications for treatment are equivocal or where there is disagreement among doctors should be made explicit. This is partly because guidelines for circulation beyond an originating group should reflect a wide measure of agreement, based if possible on published literature, about what constitutes good practice; secondly, because areas of disagreement can form the basis of future controlled trials to determine the efficacy of different treatments.

Although the examples give in this section have mainly been of secondary care procedures, the same problems relate to primary care and to hospital referrals. GPs are known to vary in their views about their responsibility for managing some conditions (Whitfield and Bucks 1988). For example, a sample of consultant dermatologists showed a marked divergence of views on the question of whether GPs should refer patients with warts to hospital (Roland and Dixon 1989). Difficulty in agreeing about clinical management, and in particular hospital referral, should be welcomed as part of a developing relationship between GPs and hospital doctors. The involvement of both groups in developing guidelines which can be used to measure the appropriateness of referrals will lead to improved understanding of the position of the other, and an improved chance of making the best use of available resources.

References

Barton, E., Gallagher, S., Flower, C.D.R., Hanka, R., King, R.H., and Sherwood, T. (1987). Influence on patient management of general practitioner direct access to radiological services. *British Journal of Radiology* **60**, 893–6.

Brook, R.H. (1990). Relationship between appropriateness and outcome. In: *Measuring the outcomes of medical care* (ed. A. Hopkins and D. Costain) Royal College of Physicians and King's Fund Centre for Health Services Development, London.

Brook, R.H., Kosecoff, J.B., Park, R.E., Chassin, M.R., Winslow, C.M., Hampton, J.R. (1988). Diagnosis and treatment of coronary disease: comparison of doctor's attitudes in the USA and the UK. *Lancet* **2**, 750–3.

Chassin, M.R., Brook, R.H., Park, R.E. *et al.* (1986). Variations in the use of medical and surgical services by the Medicare Population. *New England Journal of Medicine* **314**, 285–90.

Colquhoun, I.R., Saywell, W.R., Dewbury, K.C. (1988). An analysis of referrals for primary diagnostic abdominal ultrasound to a general X-ray department. *British Journal of Radiology* **61**, 297–300.

Coulter, A., Seagroatt, V., and McPherson, M. (1990). Relation between general practices' outpatient referral rates and rates of elective admission to hospital. *British Medical Journal* **301**, 273–6.

Coulter, A., Bradlow, J., Agass, M., Martin-Bates, C., and Tulloch, A. (1991). Outcomes of referral to gynaecology outpatient clinics for menstrual problems: an audit of general practice records. *British Journal of Obstetrics and Gynaecology* **98**, 789–96.

Eddy, D.M. (1990). Clinical decision making: from theory to practice. The Challenge. *Journal of the American Medical Association* **263**, 287–90.

Ellwood, P.M. (1988). Outcomes management: a technology of patient experience. *New England Journal of Medicine* **318**, 1549–56.

Feinstein, A. (1985). A bibliography of publications on observer variability. *Journal of Chronic Disease* **38**, 619–32.

Glover, J.A. (1938). The incidence of tonsillectomy in school children. *Proceedings of the Royal Society of Medicine* **31**, 1219–36.

Gottlieb, L.K., Margolis, C.Z., and Schoenbaum, C.S. (1990). Clinical practice guidelines at an HMO: development and implementation in a quality improvement model: *Quality Review Bulletin* **16**, 80–6.

Grace, J.F. and Armstrong, D. (1987). Referral to hospital: perceptions of patients, general practitioners and consultants about necessity and suitability of referral. *Family Practice* **14**, 170–5.

Helliwell, P.S. and Wright, V. (1991). Referrals to rheumatology. *British Medical Journal* **302**, 304–5.

Hopkins, A., Menken, M., De Friese, G.H., and Feldman, R.G. (1989). Differences in strategies and treatment of neurologic disease among British and American neurologists. *Archives of Neurology* **46**, 1142–8.

Juncosa, S., Jones, R.B., and McGhee, S.M. (1990). Appropriateness of hospital referral for hypertension. *British Medical Journal* **300**, 646–8.

Kerrigan, D.D., Brown, S.R., and Hutchinson, G.H. (1990). Open access gastroscopy: too much to swallow? *British Medical Journal* **300**, 374–6.

Knottnerus, J.A., Joosten, J., and Daams, J. (1990). Comparing the quality of referrals of general practitioners with high and average referral rates: an independent panel review. *British Journal of General Practice* **40**, 178–81.

MacArthur, C. and Smith, A. (1983). Delay in the diagnosis of colorectal cancer. *Journal of the Royal College of General Practitioners* **33**, 159–61.

Merrick, N.J., Fink, A., Park, R.E., Brook, R.H., Kosecoff, J., Chassin, M.R. *et al.* (1987). Derivation of clinical indications for carotid endarterectomy by an expert panel. *American Journal of Public Health* **77**, 187–90.

Mills, P., Joseph, A.E.A., and Adam, E.J. (1989). Total abdominal and pelvic ultrasound: incidental findings and a comparison between outpatient and general practice referrals in 1000 cases. *British Journal of Radiology* **62**, 974–6.

Mooney, G. and Andersen, T.F. (1990). Challenges facing modern health care. In *The challenges of medical practice variations* Ed. T.F. Andersen and G. Mooney. MacMillan, London.

Moss, J.G., Ross, N.B., and Small, W.P. (1984). Sources of referral and letter content of acute surgical emergencies referred to one general surgical unit. *Health Bulletin* **42**, 126–31.

Park, R.E., *et al.* (1986) Physician ratings of appropriate indications for six medical and surgical procedures. *American Journal of Public Health* **76**, 766–71.

Perrin, J.M., Homer, C.T., Berwick, D.M. *et al.* (1989). Variations in rates of hospitalisation of children in three urban communities. *New England Journal of Medicine* **320**, 1183–7.

Reynolds, D., Chitnis, J.E. and Roland, M.O. (1991). General practitioner referrals: do good doctors refer more patients to hospital. *British Medical Journal* **302**, 1250–2.

Roland, M.O. and Dixon, M. (1989). Problems in setting standards for hospital referrals: experience with warts. *British Medical Journal* **299**, 658–9.

Roland, M.O., Porter, R., Matthews, J.G., Redden, J.F., Simonds, G.W., and Bewley, B. (1991). Improving care: a study of orthopaedic outpatient referrals. *British Medical Journal* **302**, 1124–8.

Ross, A.K., Davis, W.A., Horn, G., and Williams, R. (1983). General practice orthopaedic outpatient referrals in North Staffordshire. *British Medical Journal* **287**, 1439–41.

Royal College of Physicians (1990). Report of a working group: guidelines for the management of acute urinary tract infection in childhood. *Journal of the Royal College of Physicians* **25**, 36–41.

Samantha, A. and Roy, S. (1988). Referrals from general practice to a rheumatology clinic. *British Journal of Rheumatology* **27**, 74–6.

Sanders, D., Coulter, A., and McPherson, K. (1989). Variations in hospital admission rates. King's Fund, London.

Scully, C., Malamos, D., Levers, B.G.H., Porter, S.R., and Prime, S.S. (1986). Sources and patterns of referrals of oral cancer: role of general practitioners. *British Medical Journal* **293**, 599–601.

Skrabanek, P. (1990). Nonsensus consensus. *Lancet* **1**, 1446–7.

Sladden, M.J. and Graham-Brown, R.A.C. (1989). How many GP referrals to dermatology outpatients are really necessary? *Journal of the Royal Society of Medicine* **82**, 347–8.

Smith, A. (1991). In seach of consensus: no agreement on who should write guidelines or how they should be used. *British Medical Journal* **302**, 800.

South Bedfordshire Practitioners Group (1990). Development of renal scars in children: missed opportunities in management. *British Medical Journal* **301**, 1082–4.

Springall, R.G. and Todd, I.P. (1988). General practitioner referral of patients with lower gastrointestinal symptoms. *Journal of the Royal Society of Medicine* **81**, 87–8.

Stower, M.J. (1988). Delays in diagnosing and treating bladder cancer. *British Medical Journal* **296**, 1228–9.

Tarlov, A.R., Ware, J.E., Greenfield, S., Nelson, E.C., Perrin, E.C., and Zubkoff, M. (1989). The medical outcomes study. An application of methods for monitoring the results of medical care. *Journal of the American Medical Association* **282**, 925–30.

Tredennick, H. (translated) (1969). Plato: the last days of Socrates. Penguin, London.

UK–TIA Study Group. Variation in the use of angiography and carotid endarterectomy by neurologists in the UK–TIA aspirin study. *British Medical Journal* **286**, 514–7.

Visiger, D., Apter, A., Aviram, V., and Maoz, B. (1984). Over-utilisation of the general hospital emergency room for psychiatric referrals in an Israeli hospital. *American Journal of Public Health* **74**, 73–5.

Wennberg, J.E., Freeman, J.L., and Culp, W.J. (1987). Are hospital services rationed in New Haven or over-utilised in Boston. *Lancet* **1**, 1185–9.

Whitfield, M. and Bucks, R. (1988). General Practitioners' responsibilities to their patients. *British Medical Journal* **297**, 398–400.

11 Auditing referrals

Angela Coulter

Introduction — The purpose of audit

Medical audit has been defined as 'the systematic, critical analysis of the quality of medical care, including the procedures used for diagnosis and treatment, the use of resources and the resulting outcome and quality of life for the patient' (Secretaries for State 1989). Marinker (1990) has stated that 'medical audit is nothing less than an attempt to apply scientific method to the quest for quality'.

There are three main components to the audit cycle: the development of standards or guidelines, observing practice, comparing it against the standards, and implementing change. Then one proceeds through the cycle again, reviewing the guidelines and the measurement criteria, observing practice once more and, if necessary, implementing further change. Although some audits start by developing guidelines, others enter the cycle by first undertaking systematic observations of clinical practice to obtain baseline measurements and to identify issues which should be incorporated in guidelines.

A common starting point for auditing the interface between primary and secondary care is to collect data on referral rates. Many GPs have been keen to examine their referral rates and to compare these with those of their colleagues, but few have made the transition to the next stage in the process — setting standards and developing guidelines for referral — and even fewer have closed the loop of the audit cycle.

Comparing referral rates

The comparison of referral rates is the most common point of entry to the audit process because doctors are usually interested to see how their practice patterns compare with others. If a number of practices are involved then they can start by comparing rates derived from the information in annual reports. Most studies of referral rates reveal wide variations between practices or between individual GPs. This usually stimulates interest in trying to explain the differences.

As we saw in Chapter 5, there are a number of possible explanations which should be considered. These include the possibility that the observed variations may be artefactual due to differences in the quality and completeness of the information collected, that they arise because of differences in the characteristics of the populations served, or because of differences in access to specialist services, or in the availability of facilities or special expertise in the practices.

If none of these factors can account for the differences then it is reasonable to conclude that the variations are due to differences in practice styles; i.e. GPs' decision-making procedures and patterns of care. The major implication of the research into referral patterns is that the likelihood of referral to a specialist is influenced by factors as yet unidentified, which may be quite distinct from the patient's presenting problem. In other words, faced with the same patient, different doctors would make different decisions about the need for specialist intervention.

It is important to remember that referral rates in themselves do not reveal anything very useful about the quality of care. As we have seen in Chapter 6, many studies have attempted to explain the wide differences in referral rates in relations to differential health needs in the practice populations, differences in the availability of hospital services, and differences in the experience and expertise of GPs. None of these factors appear to account for much of the variation and none of them provide any pointers to what a desirable rate of referral would be.

In the absence of a consensus about the most desirable rate of referral it is important that audit groups progress beyond simply comparing rates. Indeed, it could be argued that a focus on rates alone is harmful. An approach which is aimed at identifying and penalizing the outliers (those with high or low rates) runs the risk of alienating them and encouraging complacency in the majority. An educationally sounder approach aims to raise the level of critical awareness more generally. If this is to be achieved then it will be necessary to look at the results or outcomes of referral decisions, with the intention of searching for ways in which the process could be improved to benefit patient care.

Contrasting approaches to quality improvement

That there may be a need to improve the quality of referrals should be clear from the preceding chapters in this book. The wide variations in GPs' referral rates are indicative of a lack of consensus about the appropriate use of specialist services. This phenomenon is not restricted to general practice; wide variations have been identified in hospitalization rates for common surgical procedures and medical admissions in many western developed countries (Sanders *et al.* 1989).

These variations in health care utilization have implications for costs and for quality. They raise questions about the extent to which health care delivery is as efficient, effective, and equitable as it might be. There are two possible approaches to dealing with the phenomenon of variations in medical practice, both of which are being advocated by those concerned to improve the quality of GPs' referrals.

The first approach conceptualizes the problem as stemming from inappropriate behaviour on the part of certain doctors. The high-referring GPs refer too frequently to outpatient departments, while the low referrers do not refer frequently enough. The behaviour of those GPs who refer at the average rate is seen as unproblematic. The problem lies with the deviant outliers. The proposed solution is to feed back information to GPs on their referral rates in the hope that the high and low referrers will modify their behaviour when they see the extent to which they deviate from the mean.

The second approach focuses not on individual doctor performance but on the impact of care on particular groups of patients. This view stresses the extent of ignorance about the outcomes of specific treatments and procedures. Variation is seen as arising from a lack of consensus about when an intervention is appropriate. In order to reduce the level of uncertainty and hence the variations in health care delivery proponents of this approach aim to develop guidelines or protocols for referral based on scientific evidence of the effectiveness of medical interventions.

This second approach to auditing referrals is more demanding, but it is closer to the scientific ideal than the first. There is, of course, no sound reason for believing that the average referral rate is superior to those at either end of the spectrum, unless there is valid evidence that this is the case.

Guidelines for referral ought to be based on a thorough understanding of the referral process and the effects of treatment. They should aim to give guidance on the selection of patients for referral and on management prior to referral. There is, therefore, a need to describe the current situation in order to identify problems and potential for change. The development of referral guidelines is discussed in more detail in the following chapters. This chapter focuses on the type of information necessary to monitor the outcomes of referral decisions.

Collecting data to monitor referrals

There are two main approaches to assessing the results of referrals using routine data obtainable from patients' medical records. The first uses a numerical approach to monitor organizational issues of general applicability, such as waiting-times, and so on. The second uses case-studies to study the experience of patients with particular 'tracer' conditions and to monitor clinical outcomes. Both methods require agreement on objectives and on the selection of indicators to assess whether or not the objectives have been achieved.

Monitoring organizational issues

One of the government's aims in introducing the purchaser–provider split into NHS management (see Chapter 4) was to improve the speed and responsiveness of hospital care. At the time when Thatcher's government instituted the NHS Review there was widespread public concern about a perceived deterioration in the quality of care provided by NHS hospitals. While many saw the causes as lying in the underfunding of the NHS, the government preferred to focus on seeking out and eradicating inefficiencies in the system. An important part of the strategy was to encourage health care purchasers (DHAs and GP fundholders) to build specific quality criteria into their contracts with providers. Pioneers in the GP fundholding scheme seized the opportunity to exert some influence by developing quality targets. The following targets for outpatient referrals were developed by a group of fundholders in Oxfordshire (Stephenson 1991):

1. Appointments for new outpatients to be within 12 weeks in the first year, 9 weeks in the second year, 6 weeks in the third year.

2. Appointment letter to be sent to patient within two weeks of GP's referral letter.

3. Patients to be seen in outpatients within 1 hour of their appointment time in the first year, 30 minutes in the second year (of the contract).

4. Follow-up outpatient appointments to be made at the time of the previous appointment or sent within 5 working days.

5. No more than two outpatient follow-up appointments to be arranged without consultation with the GP.

6. Investigations to be carried out where possible on the same day as the outpatient appointment.

7. Duplication of tests, especially X-rays, to be avoided.

8. Shared protocols and continuity of care to be encouraged.

DHA were told to consult with local GPs to identify their preferred referral patterns, prior to placing contracts with hospitals and other provider units. This new strategy offered GPs an opportunity to make a direct input into health service planning, based on their knowledge of the needs of their patients. Some HAs went to considerable lengths to survey GPs' opinions about the quality criteria which should be incorporated in district contracts with hospitals. As an example, GPs in City and Hackney HA asked for a commitment that discharge slips would be received within one week of all patients leaving hospital, that all new patients would be seen by a consultant or registrar, that clinic letters would include a management plan for each patient, that consultants would answer questions raised by GPs in referral letters, and that other specified quality criteria would be complied with (Bowling *et al.* 1991).

There is little point in including quality criteria in hospital contracts unless they are routinely monitored. Until recently there were no standard minimum data sets covering communications between GPs and specialist clinics, and information was recorded in a haphazard manner. The situation is improving as recommendations on information transfer are being implemented, but the onus will remain with GPs to monitor the extent to which the targets are being met.

It is important to monitor the process of care to ensure that resources are used as efficiently as possible and that patients' needs are being met. An example of a topic which could be tackled by audit groups is the issue of repeated outpatient attendances. Many outpatient departments have long waiting-lists, not primarily because of the number of new referrals but because of the number of repeat visits by patients referred previously. There have been many suggestions that outpatient departments retain patients in their care unnecessarily. In an analysis of 260 follow-up medical outpatient consultations, Marsh (1982) concluded that a large proportion were 'a complete waste of time'. GPs reported that nothing new was learnt in 61 per cent of these follow-up consultations, and in 90 per cent the patient's management was not altered as a result of the outpatient visit.

It is often asserted that one of the major causes of continuing attendance at outpatient clinics is the failure by junior doctors to discharge patients back to the care of their GPs. A study of patients referred to rheumatology clinics provided support for this view (Sullivan and Hoare 1990). Out of the 179 referrals studied, 34 per cent of the patients with rheumatoid arthritis and 10 per cent of those with osteoarthritis made four or more visits to the clinic. The patients were twice as likely to be discharged if they saw a consultant than if they saw a junior doctor.

Implementing change in this type of situation is a complex managerial task, requiring agreement between GPs and specialists on protocols for shared care. Discussion has to occur at a local level and would depend on both parties having common objectives. The effects of earlier discharge from outpatient care on patients' well-being should be monitored. An assessment of the costs and benefits of a particular policy should also take account of the inconvenience, or otherwise, to the patient of attending the clinic. As we have seen in Chapter 9, patients' views of the need for specialist consultation often differ from those of their doctors, so they should be consulted before change is agreed.

When planning this type of organizational or process audit it is important to think about ways in which change might be implemented. There will be an increasing need for audit to cross specialty boundaries and to involve nurses, paramedical staff, and managers in multidisciplinary audit groups (Moss and Smith 1991). Further examples of organizational issues which could be topics for audit include the following:

1. Waiting times: time from referral to appointment could be measured for particular specialty clinics where a problem is suspected. Results could be discussed with hospital consultants and managers, with the aim of agreeing a strategy for improvement and a target average waiting-time plus upper limit. Re-measurement could assess the extent to which the target has been reached.

2. Attendance rates: the numbers of patients failing to attend outpatient appointments could be collected and the reasons for non-attendance ascertained by means of questionnaires to patients. Agreed changes to appointment systems could be implemented and subsequent attendance rates monitored.

3. Re-referrals and cross-referrals: the number of times that patients are re-referred to outpatient clinics or cross-referred from one specialty to another and the reasons for these referrals could be monitored, with the aim of securing improvements in the initial choice of specialist. There may be a case for GPs to be provided with regularly updated information on the expertise and interests of hospital specialists.

4. Investigations and treatments: the investigations and treatments initiated in the outpatient department can be compared with those carried out in general practice, with the aim of eliminating any duplication or inefficient use of resources.

5. Communications: referral and discharge letters could be scrutinized with a view to improving communications (see Chapter 8). It will be important to consider the amount and breadth of information required, as well as the clarity and timeliness of the communications.

6. Prescribing: arrangements for prescribing could be reviewed jointly by GPs and hospital staff and agreed guidelines monitored. This is a particularly sensitive area following the introduction of indicative prescribing budgets for GPs, at a time when pressure on hospitals to reduce costs is increasing.

7. Direct access: direct access arrangements for investigation and treatment services could be reviewed and an extension of access agreed where this seems desirable.

8. Patient satisfaction: GPs might consider organizing surveys of their patients to determine their views of the outpatient services, including such issues as in-clinic waiting-times, appointment arrangements, quality and

readability of the information provided, attitudes of staff, availability of interpreters, cleanliness of premises and waiting-room facilities. These could be planned in conjunction with community health councils or FHSAs.

Monitoring clinical outcomes

Clinical outcomes can be monitored by selecting a 'tracer' condition (a common condition or illness which is interesting for some reason, or which poses particular problems with regard to referral) and auditing the notes of all patients with this condition. The outcomes of the referral can then be assessed in relation to the GP's objectives in seeking specialist intervention.

There are a variety of reasons for referring patients to specialist outpatient clinics. In a study of referrals to outpatient clinics in the Oxford region, GPs were asked to record their main reason for each referral, as well as details about the patient, their condition, the referring hospital, and so on (Coulter *et al.* 1989). Records were kept of 18 754 referrals. The reported reasons for referral were categorized and distributed as follows:

(1) to establish the diagnosis (the diagnosis was unclear) — 28 per cent;

(2) for a specified investigation (the diagnosis was reasonably clear) — 7 per cent;

(3) for treatment or an operation (the diagnosis was known) — 35 per cent;

(4) for advice on management and referral back (the diagnosis was known) — 14 per cent;

(5) for a specialist to take over the management (the diagnosis was known) — 9 per cent;

(6) for a second opinion to reassure them (the GPs) that they had done all that was required — 2 per cent;

(7) for a second opinion to reassure patients or their families that they (the GPs) had done all that was required — 2 per cent;

(8) for other reasons — 2 per cent.

Use of this classification revealed a diverse range of referral object-ives and expectations which differed widely according to the patient's presenting condition. The situation becomes even more complex when one takes account of the fact that there is often more than one reason for referring a patient. As an example, a diagnosis or exclusion of a diagnosis may be required in order to reassure a patient, but the GP may also require advice from the specialist on the most appropriate treatment option. Specifying one main objective is not necessarily straightforward, but it helps to try to clarify reasons for referral if one is attempting to assess whether the clinical objectives have been achieved.

Referrals for diagnosis As an example, if the main reason for referral was to establish or confirm a diagnosis then one can examine whether the GP's tentative diagnosis (if there was one) concurred with the specialist's diagnosis. One could then look further to see whether clarification of a diagnosis resulted in any alteration of the patient's treatment; in other words, was a diagnosis necessary? If an investigation was specified then one could audit the notes to see if it was performed, whether or not the diagnosis was confirmed, and whether the management of the patient changed as a result.

It is often asserted that many of the diagnostic tests and investigations performed in outpatient departments are unnecessary, although it is important not to overlook the potential benefit of negative tests. Haines *et al.* (1980) looked at abnormality rates in barium meals ordered by GPs and consultants, to see whether GPs were more likely to order these inappropriately. They found no significant difference in the proportion of tests showing major abnormalities between patients referred by hospital doctors and those referred by GPs. However, they concluded that the value of this investigation could not be fully assessed merely by recording the proportion showing abnormal findings, since a normal investigation may be of great importance both for the reassurance of the patient and in diagnosis.

Sometimes the concern about unnecessary investigation stems from a worry about possible risk to the patient, rather than simply the need to promote the efficient use of resources. The use of radiological invest-igation is one such example. Halpin *et al.* (1991) studied GPs' referrals for lumbar spine radiography to see whether they complied with guidelines developed by the Royal College of Radiologists. They concluded that 52 out of 100 consecutive examinations studied should not have been requested and they were concerned that patients were being subjected to potentially harmful ionizing radiation unnecessarily.

Referrals for advice or reassurance If the main purpose of the referral was for advice on management or reassurance, with the expectation that the patient would be referred back to the GP after the consultation, one can look to see whether that advice was received, whether or not the patient was discharged after one visit, and whether or not the patient was reassured. Consultation rates before and after the referral might be used as a crude indicator of the extent to which the goal of reassurance was achieved, but this is no substitute for asking patients directly.

If the GP is expecting to receive specialist advice then it is relevant to consider whether the patient was in fact seen by an experienced specialist.

Kiff and Sykes (1988) monitored all outpatient clinics in a district general hospital for a period of four weeks; they found that less than half of all new patients were seen by a consultant. In the medical clinics just over a quarter of patients were seen by doctors who had less than six months' experience in their specialty. Consultation times were often brief and many of the patients saw tired doctors who had been on continuous duty for at least 24 hours prior to the consultation.

Referrals for treatment   If the GP expects the referral to result in the patient being given a particular treatment, or intends the specialist to take over the management of the patient for a while, the evaluation could examine whether the specialist did instigate the treatment as expected. In fact, it is often the case that the reason for referral is not specified in a referral letter. In the absence of any evidence to the contrary, specialists may assume that the GP and the patient expect a treatment to be offered, rather than just advice or reassurance.

In a study of referrals for back pain the actions initiated in the outpatient clinics were compared with the GPs' expectations recorded at the time of referral (Coulter *et al.* 1991*b*). Three quarters of the patients received treatment in the clinic, despite the fact that the GPs had recorded this as the main reason for referral in only 29 per cent of cases. Of those patients referred primarily for advice and reassurance, 69 per cent received some form of treatment in the outpatient clinic.

All of these issues may provide starting points for the development of referral guidelines, but ultimately the most important outcome is the patient's condition following referral, as compared with the likely outcome if he or she had not been referred. The application of scientific method to the referral decision requires accurate estimates of the probability of various outcomes coupled with a full understanding of patients' values and preferences (Eddy 1984; Coulter 1991). Unfortunately, scrutiny of routine case notes cannot provide the necessary information for a scientific evaluation.

The limits to audit

Most of the audit studies cited above were concerned with organizational issues or the process of care. Yet the definition of audit with which this chapter began included the assessment of the outcomes of treatment and the resulting quality of life of patients. It is important to understand the limitations of routine clinical records for assessing treatment outcomes. The following example illustrates some of the problems.

A study of the case-notes of general practice patients who had been referred to gynaecology outpatient clinics looked at the immediate results of referral and at symptom prevalence and consultation rates five years after referral (Coulter *et al.* 1991*a*). The 205 patients in the study, who were referred for menstrual disorders, received a variety of treatments for their condition: 44 per cent underwent hysterectomy; 13 per cent underwent a procedure such as curettage, IUCD removal or replacement, cervical biopsy, colposcopy, or diathermy; 12 per cent received drug therapy only; 24 per cent received a combination of drugs and procedure; and 5 per cent received no active therapy. Five years later audit of the general practice notes suggested that symptoms had resolved for the majority of women in each of the treatment groups. It is tempting to assume that all these women must therefore have been referred and treated appropriately, but this conclusion would not be warranted on the basis of the information collected in the audit.

There were three important reasons why the results could not be used to assess the appropriateness of the referral decisions. The records included no information about case-severity on which to judge the urgency of the problem and the comparability of the treatment groups; they excluded patients' subjective experiences of illness and outcomes and their treatment preferences; and for the most part they included only those patients who had received treatment, thus providing no information about the natural history of the untreated condition. These limitations are common to most medical audit studies which depend on routinely-collected data.

In order to disentangle treatment effects from the natural history of the disease it would be necessary to have a control group of patients with similar levels of symptomatology who were not treated. In order to make judgements about an appropriate rate of referral, information would also be needed on patients' preferences, since these are important in the choice of treatment for benign conditions like menorrhagia. It is rare to find such information recorded in general practice case notes.

From audit to outcomes research

While much can be learned from retrospective study of referrals and their aftermath — observation of practice being an essential step in the audit — as we have seen, such an exercise usually raises more questions than it answers. If practice guidelines are to be soundly based on scientific evidence, and if it is true that only about 15 per cent of medical interventions are supported by solid scientific evidence (Smith 1991), then audit groups have a problem. They may choose to restrict themselves to those areas where there is good evidence on which to base 'good practice' guidelines, but these may not include many of the most common reasons for referral from primary to secondary care. Alternatively, they may decide to focus on the process issues discussed earlier, avoiding the attempt to relate process to outcome. Whichever course they adopt will not preclude the need to give some attention to the scientific justification, or lack of it, for the clinical interventions they commonly use. Audit can be judged a success if it encourages awareness of the need for more controlled studies of the outcomes of illness and treatment.

The focus should move beyond the assessment of the appropriateness of referral decisions to a more far-reaching assessment of the effectiveness of different forms of treatment and patterns of care. The aim would be to build a consensus on when particular medical interventions are appropriate, based on an understanding of clinical outcomes, together with patients' evaluations of their symptoms and quality of life before and after treatment. Patients should not be referred for treatments which are not likely to be effective.

In many ways general practice offers an excellent base for research into the outcomes of health care; the existence of complete clinical records enables an examination of the antecedents and duration of a particular illness episode and patients can be followed up over a long period of time. Ideally, outcomes studies require random allocation of patients to the different groups under comparison. There is no reason why such studies should not be initiated in general practice, although these will go beyond the scope of medical audit as it is currently practised and resourced. However, it is probable that the distinction between medical audit and health services research will increasingly become blurred. If the critical approach advocated here is adopted more widely in general practice audit then it should stimulate awareness of the need for more research, and hopefully GPs will be encouraged to get involved. It is to be hoped that many more randomized controlled trials will be established to settle some of the uncertainty surrounding referral decisions. The main task of audit will then be to ensure that the results of the research are applied in clinical practice.

Auditing the audit

The audit process itself should be the subject of audit. Projects which fail to demonstrate an improvement in the quality of care should be critically examined to see why they have failed. Audit of routine data is an excellent means of monitoring the referral process and the speed and quality of service offered to GPs and their patients by hospital departments, but true improvements in health status will require more than this.

The North of England study of standards and performance in general practice (Centre for Health Services Research 1991) provides a model for the way in which audit can be evaluated. By using a 'Latin-square' design they were able to evaluate the effect of five different approaches:

(1) active involvement in setting a clinical standard;

(2) receiving a copy of a clinical standard set by another group;

(3) receiving comparative feedback showing their performance as compared with the performance of others;

(4) receiving feedback on their performance alone;

(5) no intervention.

Only those doctors actively involved in standard-setting demonstrated a subsequent change in their clinical behaviour. This is an important finding because it reinforces the argument that passive receipt of externally-developed guidelines is unlikely to be effective unless accompanied by additional incentives to change (Chapter 13).

Even more importantly, this study attempted to assess the effect of audit on patients' health status. It was only possible to demonstrate an effect for one of the five paediatric conditions studied; recurrent wheezy chest. Following the development of guidelines there was a change in prescribing patterns for this condition. Antibiotics were replaced by different drug therapies, resulting in a 50p increase in the average annual drug cost per child, and better compliance with drug therapy. There was evidence of more follow-up care with an increased number of doctor-initiated consultations. This increase in resource use resulted in an average reduction of 3 days per month in the number of days in which parents reported their children were breathless, and a reduction of 3.6 days per month when the children were wheezy.

Those involved in clinical audit should strive to evaluate their efforts in terms of the effect on patient outcomes. The North of England study confirmed that this will require more sophisticated information systems than routine medical records. They used structured records, home interviews, postal outcome questionnaires, GP surveys, surgery records, and practice activity records. The study authors also argued that successful audit requires educational skills, training in small group leadership, external review, research skills, and resources for literature review.

Conclusion

The need for scientific assessment of health care interventions, on which all guidelines should be based, is as pressing as ever. Audit should be the means of ensuring that the results of scientific evaluation are applied in clinical practice. Where the necessary scientific evidence does not exist because evaluative studies have not been carried out, audit can help to raise questions about the best form of clinical care, but it will not provide the answers.

References

Bowling, A., Jacobsen, B., Southgate, L., and Formby, J. (1991). General practitioners' views on quality specifications for 'outpatient referrals and care contracts'. *British Medical Journal* **303**, 292–4.

Centre for Health Services Research Ambulatory Care Programme (1991). *North of England study of standards and performance in general practice. Department of Health, London.*

Coulter, A. (1991). Evaluating the outcomes of health care. In *The sociology of the health service* (ed. J. Gabe, M. Calnan, and M. Bury). Routledge, London.

Coulter, A., Bradlow, J., Agass, M., Martin-Bates, C., and Tulloch, A. (1991*a*) Outcomes of referrals to gynaecology outpatient clinics for menstrual problems: an audit of general practice records. *British Journal of Obstetrics and Gynaecology* **98**, 789–96.

Coulter, A., Bradlow, J., Martin-Bates, C., Agass, M., and Tulloch, A. (1991*b*). What happens to patients referred to specialist outpatient clinics for back pain? *British Journal of General Practice* **41**, 450–3.

Coulter, A., Noone, A., and Goldacre, M. (1989). General practitioners' referrals to specialist outpatient clinics. *British Medical Journal* **299**, 304–8.

Eddy, D.M. (1984). Variations in physician practice: the role of uncertainty. *Health Affairs* **3**, 74–89.

Haines, A., Ashleigh, R., Bates, R., and Kreel, L. (1980). The use of barium meals by general practitioners and hospital doctors. *Journal of the Royal Collage of General Practitioners* **30**, 97–100.

Halpin, S., Yeoman, L., and Dundas, D. (1991). Radiographic examination of the lumber spine in a community hospital: an audit of current practice. *British Medical Journal* **303**, 813–5.

Kiff, R.S. and Sykes, P.A. (1988). Who undertakes the consultations in the outpatient department? *British Medical Journal* **296**, 1511–2.

Marinker, M. (ed) (1990). *Medical audit and general practice* MSD Foundation/ British Medical Journal, London.

Marsh, G.N. (1982). Are follow-up consultations at medical outpatient departments futile? *British Medical Journal* **284**, 1176–7.

Moss, F. and Smith, R. (1991). From audit to quality and beyond. *British Medical Journal* **303**, 199–200.

Sanders, D., Coulter, A., and McPherson, K. (1989). *Variations in hospital admission rates: a review of the literature.* King's Fund, London.

Secretaries of State for Social Services, Wales, Northern Ireland and Scotland (1989). *Working for patients.* HMSO (Cm 555), London.

Smith, R. (1991). Where is the wisdom . . . . .? *British Medical Journal* **303**, 798–9.

Stephenson, R. (1991). GP fund-holding: a spirit of optimism. *Primary Health Care Management* **1** (8), 5–6.

Sullivan, F. and Hoare, T. (1990). New referrals to rheumatology clinics — why do they keep coming back? *British Journal of Rheumatology* **29**, 53–7.

12 Developing referral guidelines

Andrew Haines and David Armstrong

Introduction

Traditionally GPs have guarded their claim to clinical autonomy so that clinical decisions could be made in the best interests of each individual patient. However, in recent years the idea of introducing some sort of external referrent for such decisions has become common in medicine. In part this has arisen because of the increased complexity of medical decision-making and a rapid expansion of diagnostic and therapeutic capabilities. There also is an increasing recognition of the wide range of medical responses to specific conditions which, in the context of an increasing awareness of the need to use limited resources in the most cost-effective manner, has provided an added impetus to the development of mechanisms for influencing clinical management decisions.

Three ways of exerting influence on a doctor's decision-making have been identified by Eddy (1990a): these are standards, guidelines, and options. Standards are intended to be applied rigidly and are appropriate in situations in which exceptions to the rules are unusual and violation constitutes poor medical practice. Arguably such situations are few in general practice. Guidelines are more flexible and although they should be followed in most cases, they must be tailored to fit individual needs. Deviations from the guidelines by themselves do not imply incompetence. In order to compile a guideline, at least a number of the important outcomes of a given intervention must be known. Topics on which such information is not available, or where the evidence indicates several equally effective courses of action, generate options.

There are a variety of different ways of constructing guidelines (Eddy 1990b) but they have in common the broad aims of improving clinical management of a condition (including diagnosis, treatment, referral, discharge, and patient knowledge) and facilitating more cost-effective use of limited resources. In addition, guidelines may promote closer working relationships between GPs and specialists if they are drawn up in a way which emphasizes the appropriate contributions of both parties. They can also provide standards for performance review and fulfill an important educational function.

There is now considerable experience available in the setting of, using, and evaluating clinical guidelines. Most of these examples relate to aspects of hospital medicine (for example, Fowkes *et al.* 1986, 1987; Hall *et al.* 1988; Roberts *et al.* 1983; Roberts 1988; Royal College of Radiologists Working Party 1981, 1983, 1985) though there have been some studies based in general practice. As an example, a considerable amount of work has been undertaken on the development of formularies which aim to promote the use of a limited range of drugs with which the practitioner can become familiar and which are cost-effective and sufficient in scope to deal with the common conditions found in general practice (Beardon *et al.* 1987; Harding *et al.* 1985). In Sweden national guidelines have been agreed for the continuing education of GPs about drugs. The guidelines recommend acquisition of very detailed knowledge of the most commonly used drugs (around 50) and familiarity with a further 150 or so drugs used somewhat less frequently (Block and Svender 1986; McGavock 1990).

The College of General Practitioners in the Netherlands has initiated a national programme to set standards for the quality of care in general practice (Grol 1990). Small working groups of 4 or 5 experienced practitioners and researchers write a draft of each set of standards and these are then circulated for comments to 50 GPs. The standards are published in the National Journal for General Practitioners (Huisarts and Wetenschap) and the main features are summarized on a plastic card sent with the Journal. A survey of a random 10 per cent sample of Dutch doctors indicated that around 70 per cent were well informed about the standards. In general there was a positive response to the setting of national standards, but fewer were actually working to them. When asked about the specific recommendations for the care of diabetes, for instance, only 33 per cent were using special diabetes records or marking practice records of diabetic patients.

The impetus for guideline development in the USA is somewhat different from that in Europe, and relates to the desire of government and insurance companies to limit spiralling costs and perceived overutilization of health care resources. Current efforts in America centre around attempts to produce guidelines which are based on scientific evidence of what constitutes effective, and cost-effective, medical treatment. The Agency for Health Care Policy and Research (AHCPR) was established in 1989 by the government with responsibility for producing scientifically valid clinical guidelines. The approach of the AHCPR is to produce a decision tree for the management of a specified condition, and then to carry out an exhaustive literature review followed by meta-analysis of relevant papers in order to estimate the likely outcomes of different courses of action. Between 5000 and 75 000 (in the case of the guideline on depression in primary care) papers are included in the literature review, of which approximately 500 are sent for expert peer review. The cost of this process runs to several million dollars per guideline, and it remains to be seen whether the effort will be reflected in more appropriate use of health care resources.

European initiatives have tended to use expert or consensus groups, backed by relatively limited literature review. A number of specialty associations in the UK have recently issued guidelines, including those on asthma by the British Thoracic Society (1990) and on hyperlipidaemia by the British Hyperlipidaemia Association (Betteridge *et al.* 1987). In the case of the asthma guidelines, they include indications for referral. Guidelines from specialty associations can be useful, particularly if they are put together by a group representing the range of disciplines involved in management, or if the specialty concerned (such as in the case of radiology) is potentially in a position to control access to a particular category of investigation, and can therefore exert considerable influence on colleagues to encourage the most efficient use of resources.

One problem with 'expert'-derived guidelines is that their representativeness and applicability may be open to doubt. For many clinical procedures there is a broad range of options and often experts themselves cannot agree. This means that particular groups of experts may by chance or design under-represent the diversity of clinical opinion and thereby produce 'biased' guidelines. Also, the expert groupings often fail to invite GPs — or if they do so, involve GPs with atypical practices — and their advice may fail to take into account the practical difficulties of implementation by a non-specialist and the competing claims for improvements in care in other areas.

Some attempt has been made to overcome the unrepresentativeness of a particular expert committee by setting up a 'consensus conference' in which the experts are required to present their views to a 'jury' composed of people representing the variety of interests which might make use of the information. There have been a number of consensus statements both in North America and Europe which have laid down guidelines for specific medical conditions. As an example, the National Institutes of Health (NIH) created a Consensus Development Program to conduct public evaluation of scientific information about biomedical technologies. Consensus statements containing recommendations for medical practice have been produced on a wide range of areas including diagnosis, treatment, and prevention (Kosecoff *et al.* 1987).

Despite these attempts to widen the range of experts consulted on the setting of particular guidelines, expert opinion tends to remain an outside view from the perspective of the ordinary GP. Indeed, in many ways, GPs as independent contractors have traditionally been suspicious of outside interference; it is their business they are running, in their way, with their methods. This means that it is important for the process of developing guidelines to involve GPs and take such a form as to give GPs a sense of ownership. Ideally, for full commitment and ownership every GP should construct their own guidelines; however, such a policy simply reproduces the variation of many idiosyncratic clinical judgements without the important tempering of other professional opinion. The task therefore, on the one hand, is to involve individual GPs to such an extent that they feel they are committed to the guidelines and yet, at the same time, ensure the involvement of many GPs in their creation to ensure that they represent an optimal clinical result.

Hospital referrals would appear to be good subjects for clinical guidelines both because of their apparent variability and the high costs associated with them. Several studies have documented large variations in the rate of hospital referral by GPs which cannot be explained by the characteristics of patients, the list size, age or training of the general practitioner (Chapter 6).

Tensions in developing referral guidelines

Currently, the decision to refer a patient to hospital outpatients for advice or treatment is taken by the GP and based on the needs of the patient. This decision is an individual one and there are grounds for supposing, as indicated by other chapters in this volume, that presented with the same patient and the same context different GPs would often act differently. This variation in clinical practice between different GPs means that some patients may not be receiving care from which they might benefit whilst others are receiving treatment that is unnecessary and wasteful of expensive hospital resources. Various strategies for addressing this problem have been suggested, ranging from the coercive to the persuasive, but there are two major difficulties in trying to get GPs to change their referral habits. Firstly, in many instances it is not at all obvious what the 'correct' referral decision should be, so it is difficult to be too prescriptive about what should happen. Secondly, it is not clear which is the most effective method to persuade GPs to change their clinical practice.

The use of clinical guidelines offers one approach to trying to encourage 'good practice' in the area of hospital referrals. However, there can be important tensions between ensuring that guidelines are correct and at the same time persuasive. At one extreme the correctness of guidelines can be ensured by incorporating expert opinion (as discussed above), but this means that GPs, as non-experts, are not involved in their production and are therefore less than likely to be persuaded of their usefulness. At the other extreme GPs could be wholly involved with developing the guidelines, so ensuring ownership and commitment, yet produce something which was clearly inappropriate. This tension can be illustrated through two separate initiatives in the development of clinical guidelines for common conditions in general practice, most of which had significant advice on the appropriateness of hospital referral.

Bromley guidelines project

The development of clinical guidelines in the Bromley Health District started with the premise that all GPs in the District should have the opportunity to contribute to the development of the guidelines. In other words, the production of local guidelines was to involve those GPs who would be likely to use them. There are various formal techniques available which can be used to involve large numbers of clinicians. Perhaps the msot well known is the Delphi technique in which draft guidelines would be circulated to GPs for their comment, their comments incorporated into revised guidelines, which would again be sent out for further comment. This process continues until the best consensus is achieved, though in practice it has been found that two or three circuits is about all the respondents will support.

A variation of such techniques was used in Bromley to draw up a series of clinical guidelines for local GPs, many of which embrace referral advice. Broadly, the technique was to draw up a draft of some clinical guidelines for a particular clinical condition using a working party composed of local GPs and interested hospital consultants. These draft guidelines, in representing an agreed statement between some local GPs and consultants, had some merit in themselves and might have been sent out to local GPs in that state. However, it was clear that the GPs participating in the working party represented a very narrow cross-section of the wide range of GP opinion across the HA. The next stage was therefore to turn the draft guidelines into a questionnaire which was then sent to all GPs within the health district. Basically, the questionnaire asked the responding GP for their views on the clinical advice laid down in the guidelines. Different questionnaires experimented with different styles and the evolution of the approach over four sets of guidelines will be briefly described.

Antenatal Care   A group of local obstetricians and GPs drew together some guidelines for the management of various antenatal problems. The draft document simply offered advice on what to do in certain clinical situations. However, it was apparent that some of the advice would require GPs to alter their existing clinical practice, and would therefore need further justification; but which pieces of advice would need stressing? The way to find out was to send a questionnaire to the 160 GPs in the area to enquire about their customary clinical practice with respect to the problems identified in the draft guidelines. In this way those drafting the guidelines could take account of local variation; for example, if all GPs currently followed some recommended clinical policy then it was of little value incorporating it into the guidelines. On the other hand, if GPs showed a wide range of clinical opinion on a particular matter then

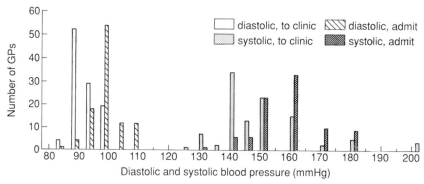

Fig. 12.1 Hypertension in pregnancy: when do GPs refer?

it was open for the drafting working party to amend the draft guidelines to explain further and justify the clinical advice which it was known would fly in the face of current practice.

As an example, the draft guidelines for hypertension in pregnancy advised referral to the next clinic if blood pressure rose as high as 90 mmHg diastolic or 140 mmHg systolic, and admission if the blood pressure rose to 100 mmHg diastolic or 140 mmHg systolic. The range of GP views is given in Fig. 12.1. GPs showed great variation, but tended to be more permissive than the working party. In the light of this the working party were invited to change their advice for the final guidelines. After much discussion, especially under the influence of the obstetricians who had agreed that the guidelines should also apply to hospital obstetric practice throughout the district, the draft advice remained unchanged for this particular item, but the opportunity was taken to send the results of the survey to GPs with their copy of the final guidelines.

Diabetes guidelines   A later set of guidelines on the management of diabetes was put together by the District's diabetologist and some local GPs. On this occasion the draft guidelines were broken into separate paragraphs and incorporated into a questionnaire. GPs were then asked for each paragraph whether or not they would agree with the recommendations. If they disagreed they were invited to comment.

This method produced a 'vote' on each item in the draft guidelines together with a varied and rich commentary on each piece of advice. As an example, advice on referring newly diagnosed diabetics to the hospital diabetes centre for 'shared care' was criticized for its assumption that in practice 'shared' only meant sharing the patient, not decisions about the management . These various comments were then collated and given to the working party for them to take account of in their final revisions to the guidelines. This strategy proved a more direct method of establishing which of the recommendations would be widely supported and which opposed so that the working party could take these factors into account in drawing up the final guidelines.

Rheumatology guidelines Production of guidelines, even in the full knowledge of likely 'support' and 'resistance' in the health district, still depended on having a definitive solution to clinical management problems. But if most GPs opposed a certain clinical policy what authority did the working party have to impose or even suggest an alternative as district-wide policy? Indeed, practically, it was unlikely that GPs would be dissuaded from their current policy even with careful justification for the new management regime.

The set of guidelines developed for the management of common rheumatological conditions recognized that a single answer was not necessarily 'politically' possible for many clinical problems and that fundamentally, if guidelines were about inducing change in behaviour, they were instruments of education. It was therefore important to accept that all views had some validity and individual clinicians were unlikely to change radically their clinical policy without time for reflection and discussion.

The draft clinical guidelines on rheumatology, constructed by a consultant rheumatologist with the support of a small group of local GPs, was therefore turned into a series of clinical vignettes in a questionnaire. The responding GPs in the district were invited to select from an accompanying list of possible management decisions which they would choose when faced by such a patient. These responses were collated and the consultant rheumatologist wrote a brief commentary on the findings before returning them to the GPs. Table 12.1 provides an example. In effect, local GPs then received a document showing the variety of local clinical opinion together with that of their local rheumatologist. The individual GP could therefore compare his or her clinical practice with that of his or her colleagues and the local consultant. Such an approach did not present guidelines as a final polished instruction but, rather, opened the way for the individual GP to reflect on these differences and to bring about local discussion and possible change of clinical management as a result.

Asthma guidelines The final set of guidelines pursued a similar pattern. These were for the management of asthma in which much of the advice involved recommendations on when to refer to hospital. Again the guidelines were drawn up by a small working party consisting of local consultants and GPs. Each statement in the guidelines was then abstracted and placed into a questionnaire with a choice of three responses; these were that the recommendation was so obvious that it did not merit

Table 12.1 *Views on the management of some localized rheumatological problems*

Problem 1: A 30-year-old woman with a one-week history of neck pain and no neurological symptoms or signs and no evidence of systemic disease.

	% of GPs answering yes
(1) Treatment with simple analgesics	79
(2) Treatment with NSAID's	40
(3) Referral for physiotherapy	5
(4) Wearing a soft cervical support collar	15
(5) X-ray	1
(6) Blood test (FBC, ESR rheumatoid factor)	2
(7) Refer to consultant rheumatologist	0
(8) None of these	6

Rheumatologist's view: Most respondents prescribed analgesics or NSAIDs. Patients with acute neck pain may be helped by physiotherapy.

Problem 2: A 60-year-old man with a history of neck pain for two years and a recent history of leg weakness.

(1) Treatment with simple analgesics	28
(2) Treatment with NSAID's	21
(3) Referral for physiotherapy	0
(4) Wearing a soft cervical support collar	17
(5) X-ray	89
(6) Blood test (FBC, ESR rheumatoid factor)	53
(7) Refer to consultant rheumatologist	34
(8) None of these	7

Rheumatologist's view: The possibility of cervical myelopathy should be considered. X-ray of the cervical spine will be necessary. The patient should be referred to a rheumatologist.

Problem 3: A 40-year-old man with a three-week history of neck pain and general ill health.

(1) Treatment with simple analgesics	51
(2) Treatment with NSAID's	21
(3) Referral for physiotherapy	1
(4) Wearing a soft cervical support collar	10
(5) X-ray	74
(6) Blood test (FBC, ESR rheumatoid factor)	94
(7) Refer to consultant rheumatologist	12
(8) None of these	3

Rheumatologist's view: The possibility of osteomyelitis should be considered. X-ray and blood tests will be necessary. The patient should be referred to a rheumatologist or orthopaedic surgeon.

Table 12.2 *The value of guidelines on the management of asthma*

---

1. **Children with an asthmatic attack who fail to respond to nebulized B2 stimulant or relapse within 4 hours of a dose should be hospitalized.**

	percentage
Obvious	51.0
Useful	38.5
Controversial	10.0

Valid cases: 96

2. **Asthmatics referred to hospital outpatients should, in general, have previously had a chest X-ray.**

	percentage
Obvious	20.8
Useful	28.1
Controversial	51.0

3. **Asthmatics referred to hospital out-patients should, in general, have had a full blood count and eosinophil count.**

	percentage
Obvious	16.7
Useful	42.7
Controversial	40.0

4. **Oral steroids should only be given to an asthmatic on a regular basis in consultation with a chest physician.**

	percentage
Obvious	16.7
Useful	28.1
Controversial	55.0

5. **In children, cyanosis during an asthma attack is indication for hospitalization.**

	percentage
Obvious	87.5
Useful	12.0
Controversial	0.0

---

inclusion in the guidelines, that it was so controversial that the particular GP would not follow it even if it were in the guidelines, and those suggestion which GPs felt would be helpful. Thus, on return of the questionnaire and collation of the results each specific recommendation in the original guidelines was accompanied by the advice of local GPs as to whether it was useful, controversial, or obvious. Table 12.2 provides an example of the material returned by GPs.

Again, rather than the 'expert' working party drawing the threads into their personal summary, the collated results were sent back to GPs in their 'raw' state. This meant that local GPs could see the wide range of clinical views of their colleagues, especially on what they thought was clinically obvious, useful, and controversial, and again the hope was that such information would prove useful in guiding individual reflection and group discussion within the district.

In summary, the Bromley clinical guideline experiment started with the intention of establishing, through high GP involvement, a set of definitive district-wide guidelines on the management of some common clinical conditions which would be widely supported. It evolved into a recognition that it was impossible to produce a document which either reflected the diversity of clinical practice or, more important, was likely to change established patterns of behaviour. There is sufficient evidence to suggest that changing clinical decision-making is a very difficult task and simply providing a list of instructions or recommendations, it was felt, would be unlikely to persuade anyone. The strategy finally adopted was therefore an educational one.

Children are traditionally taught by didactic techniques in which they are told what the answer is; adults learn by other methods, particularly by problem-solving, experience, and discussion. The Bromley experiment therefore tried to encourage this adult-learning approach by providing a rich source of data on clinical guidelines, including those on referral practice.

Islington guidelines project

This project has a somewhat different history and approach from the Bromley experiment but has also come to focus particularly on the educational component of guidelines. Its initial objectives were to harmonize management between hospital and community, to improve communication between the two, and to provide a basis for audit exercises. Topics were selected according to their prevalence, based on figures from the National Morbidity Survey (RCGP/OPCS/DHSS 1986). They were well-defined conditions that were responsible for 10 or more consultations per thousand patients in general practice. In addition, some areas of prevention, such as cervical cytology and cardiovascular prevention, were selected because of their relevance to the general practitioner contract. A few other topics such as drug misuse were added because they cause particular problems to GPs in inner city areas.

A meeting was convened to bring together GPs with local consultants. Many, but not all of the GPs, had links with the academic department of primary health care of University College and Middlesex School of Medicine. For each topic a GP and a consultant were identified and took responsibility for writing a first draft. This was circulated to a number of colleagues and, where relevant, other health professionals such as dietitians and pharmacists were also consulted. The intention was to make the guidelines evidence-based as far as possible, but exhaustive literature reviews were not undertaken because of limitations in resources. The patients perspective was included by reference to self-help and special interest groups where relevant.

Although, in general, getting an agreement on the guidelines was a relatively smooth process, it was also a time-consuming one, particularly as several topics were being considered at the same time. One difficulty which needs to be acknowledged and discussed at the outset is the difference in perspective between specialists and GPs; they see different populations of patients. GPs may sometimes be sceptical about the need to include, for instance, indications for referral and investigation, of what for them are relatively rare complications or causative factors. Specialists on the other hand may see considerable numbers of patients of this kind. These problems are often best clarified in an open meeting to discuss the guidelines. We have therefore included presentation of the guidelines jointly by a specialist and a GP in the continuing medical education programme of the local postgraduate centre. These meetings have generally been popular and have the added benefit of giving local publicity to the venture, as well as encouraging critical debate of the content of the guidelines. Another factor which needed to be taken into account was the production of national guidelines by a number of authorities during the period that the local guidelines were being compiled. Examples include the British Hyperlipidaemia Association (Betteridge *et al.* 1987), the British Thoracic Society (British Thoracic Society 1990), and the Joint Working Party on Child Health Surveillance (Hall 1989).

Another problem which arose resulted from the range of interests and competences amongst GPs in relation to specific topics. Child health surveillance is one example of this. Although a considerable number of practices undertake their own child health surveillance programmes and are eligible for payments by the FHSA, others do not, so after considerable discussion it was decided to divide the guidelines on child health surveillance into two parts. The first part comprised guidelines for all GPs, giving a brief outline of average developmental progress and a summary of the assessments at six weeks, eight months, 21 months, and 39 months. The second part was more detailed and was directed specifically to those carrying out child health surveillance clinics in the practice. These gave much more detailed indications of how to undertake surveillance. In the initial enthusiasm we planned to undertake guidelines for a larger number of topics. During the course of the project, however, it became apparent that it was more important to concentrate on a number of topics in a more focused way, rather than to spread the net too widely in the first instance. In the case of some topics there was also the difficulty of finding GPs with a particular interest in the area. It could be argued, of course, that a special interest in the area may actually be counter-productive and that the guidelines produced may be unrealistic and not applicable to the majority of GPs. A counter argument is that a GP with a special interest in a topic and a grasp of the literature may be in a better position to question assertions for which there is no adequate evidence.

A further question concerns the degree to which purchaser and provider relationships will affect the development of guidelines on referral and management. Clearly, guidelines could fit into this process, particularly from the perspective of the purchaser, whose responsibility it is to ensure that high quality care is given at the lowest possible cost.

There are a number of possible formats for guidelines ranging from very brief documents of one page or less to longer articles of several thousand words. Clearly, very brief documents can be rapidly consulted by busy doctors, but may fail to provide sufficient detail. In Islington it was decided to aim for documents of up to 2000 words in length which discussed briefly the following aspects of patient care; assessment and investigation, pharmacological and non-pharmacological treatment, indications for referral to a specialist and discharge, arrangements for follow-up and monitoring, information for patients and relatives. Any detailed technical information such as dietary advice or information about local services was listed in the form of appendices, as were telephone numbers and contact addresses for self-help and special interest groups. Subsequently, it was decided to provide a one page summary and four or five audit points which could be used by practitioners to audit their performance.

Guidelines have been completed and circulated by the FHSA to local GPs on 15 topics; hypertension, chronic heart failure, diabetes, irritable bowel syndrome, asthma, chronic obstructive airways disease, common skin conditions, back pain, heavy drinking, drug misuse, the red eye, cervical cytology, cardiovascular prevention, dementia in old age, and child health surveillance. Evaluation forms have been included with each individual guideline and these have identified a small number of specific problems, which in a few instances have resulted in additions or amendments. Devising, circulating, and discussing guidelines are only preliminary steps toward their implementation. With the advent of medical audit advisory groups and the provision of some financial backing for audit, it has now become possible for the first time to develop local strategies for the implementation and monitoring of guidelines. It is only after this that it will be possible to determine whether they have the potential to make an impact on patterns of care in everyday practice.

Other UK initiatives

There are a range of other initiatives in this country; the following is by no means an exhaustive list, but does give a flavour of early activities in this field. The RCGP itself has published folders on a range of clinical topics, edited by Colin Waine (Royal College of General Practitioners). A study of protocols for the management of chronic disease (diabetes, asthma, and hypertension) comparing nurse and GP performance is being undertaken by the Department of General Practice at Nottingham. Diabetes is also the subject of a project co-ordinated by the Department of General Practice at the University of Wales, involving a nurse facilitator. The Department of Community Medicine of the Haringey Health Authority has established a post of Primary Health Care Development Co-ordinator and developed protocols on three conditions, namely: childhood asthma, chronic rheumatological disorders, and haemoglobinopathies. The Department of Primary Medical Care at the University of Southampton has studied the resource implications of developing and introducing clinical management plans for care of patients with dyspepsia, and an experiment in shared care of epilepsy has been undertaken in Doncaster (Dennis 1989). The 'Pink Book' written by practitioners in N. Somerset has been in use for sometime (Rivett 1988). Thus there is a profusion of different initiatives currently underway.

A series of guidelines for referral has been developed in Cambridge after consultation between local GPs and specialists. In a study to determine how completely these guidelines covered the routine work of a GP, 21 GPs recorded whether patients seen over a 2-week period presented with conditions which were described by one of 64 guidelines covering 9 subject areas (each GP recorded details of three subject areas). It was estimated that the 64 guidelines covered only 14 per cent of patients seen during this period (Fertig and Roland, personal communication). This emphasizes the vast range of conditions seen by GPs and the consequent difficulty in providing guidelines to cover even a small proportion of their work.

Conclusion

Guidelines can be seen as part of the overall dynamic process of medical audit (Chapter 11). As such, guidelines should be regularly reviewed and adapted in response to advances in knowledge and changes in the organization of care. They can focus on one part of the process of diagnosis and treatment, such as referral to a hospital, or can encompass a number of key aspects of patient management. They can range from very brief statements of one page or less to documents of considerable length. It is likely, however, that if they are to be widely used they will need to be succinct and rapidly accessible in the form of a desktop guide to practice, perhaps backed up by longer reference documents. In future they may well be incorporated into general practice and hospital computer systems. Some will include algorithms which illustrate pathways of decision making.

Thus the main role of guidelines at the present time is probably educational. As greater resources are put into audit, they should become more widely used. The resources involved in devising and keeping guidelines up-to-date are considerable and there is therefore likely to be continuing debate about whether they should be generated centrally from colleges or specialist organisations or peripherally by practitioners on the 'front line'. In practice, a combination of approaches is likely, with local practitioners adapting national documents to their own requirements. At the moment, however, more work is needed to ensure that guidelines do have a measurable impact on the quality of care. In particular, more work is needed on measuring the outcomes of different clinical policies; for example, in the UK, the Standing Medical Advisory Committee has calculated the cost effectiveness of plasma cholesterol screening (Standing Medical Advisory Committee 1990), but in most cases adequate outcome measures are not available or insufficiently validated, though they are currently the subject of much research and development.

The work described in this chapter suggests that guidelines may have a useful role in stimulating discussion between specialists and GPs. Some of the problems of developing referral guidelines are similar to guidelines developed for hospital doctors, but some problems relate specifically to general practice. In the next chapter, Russell and Grimshaw consider the evidence from studies which have attempted to determine whether and under what circumstances guidelines are likely to alter clinical behaviour.

References

Beardon, P.H.G. *et al.* (1987). Introducing a drug formulary to general practice — effect on practice costs. *Journal of the Royal College of General Practitioners* **37**, 305–7.

Betteridge, D.J. *et al.* (1987). Strategies for reducing coronary heart disease and desirable limits for blood lipid concentrations: guidelines of the British Hyperlipidaemia Association. *British Medical Journal* **295**, 1245–6.

Block, I. and Svender, O. (1986). Guidelines for continuing drug education for general practitioners in Sweden. *Lakartidningen* **83**, 666–7.

British Thoracic Society, Research Unit of the Royal College of Physicians of London, King's Fund Centre, National Asthma Campaign. (1990). Guidelines for management of asthma in adults: II — acute severe asthma. *British Medical Journal* **301**, 797–800.

British Thoracic Society, Research Unit of the Royal College of Physicians of London, King's Fund Centre, National Asthma Campaign. (1990). Guidelines for management of asthma in adults: I — chronic persistent asthma. *British Medical Journal* **301**, 651–3.

Dennis, N. (1989). Primary health care development fund projects. *Progress report for the King's Fund London Project Executive Committee*. Paper C, June 1989, King's Fund Centre.

Eddy, D.M. (1990*a*). Practice policies: where do they come from? *Journal of the American Medical Association* **263**, 1265–75.

Eddy, D.M. (1990*b*). Designing a practice policy; standards, guidelines and options. *Journal of the American Medical Association* **263**, 3077–84.

Fowkes, F.G.R. *et al.* (1987). Compliance with the Royal College of Radiologists guidelines on the use of pre-operative chest radiographs. *Clinical Radiology* **38**, 45–8.

Fowkes, F.G.R. *et al.* (1986). Multicentre trial of four strategies to reduce use of a radiological test. *Lancet* **i**, 367–70.

Goldman, L. (1990) Changing physicians' behaviour. *New England Journal of Medicine* **322**, 1524–5.

Grol, R. (1990). National standard setting for quality of care in general practice: attitudes of general practitioners and response to a set of standards. *British Journal of General Practice* **40**, 361–4.

Hall, R. *et al.* (1988). The impact of guidelines in clinical outpatient practice. *Journal of the Royal College of Physicians of London* **22**, 244–7.

Harding, J.M., Modell, M., and Freudenberg, S. (1985). Prescribing: the power to set limits. *British Medical Journal* **290**, 450–3.

Kosecoff, J. *et al.* (1987). Effects of the national institutes of health consensus development program on physician practice. *Journal of the American Medical Association* **258**, 2708–13.

McGavock, H. (1990) Promoting rational therapeutics: the Swedish guidelines and a UK response. *British Journal of General Practice* **40**, 1–3.

Rees, P.J. (1990). Guidelines for the management of asthma in adults. *British Medical Journal* **301**, 771–2.

Rivett, B. (1987) *The Pink Book, a handbook for West Somerset GPs*. Somerset Health Authority and Somerset Postgraduate Centre revised 1988.

Roberts, C.J., Fowkes, F.G.R., Ennis, W.P., and Mitchell, M.W. (1983). Possible impact of audit on chest X-ray requests from surgical wards. *Lancet* **ii**, 446–8.

Roberts, C.J. (1988). Annotation: towards the more effective use of diagnostic radiology: a review of the work of the Royal College of Radiologists Working Party on the more effective use of diagnostic radiology, 1976 to 1986. *Clinical Radiology* **39**, 3–6.

Royal College of General Practitioners Office of Population Censuses and Surveys, Department of Health and Social Security. (1986). *1981–1982 morbidity statistics from general practice*, Series MB5, No 1. Her Majesty's Stationery Office, London.

Royal College of Radiologists Working Party. (1985). Head injuries in adults. *Lancet* **ii**, 1882–3.

Royal College of Radiologists Working Party. (1981). Costs and benefits of skull radiology for head injury. *Lancet* **ii**, 791–5.

Royal College of Radiologists Working Party. (1983). Patient selection for skull radiology in uncomplicated head injury. *Lancet* **i**, 115–8.

Sheldon, M.G. (1982). *Medical audit in general practice*. Occasional paper 20, Royal College of General Practitioners, London.

Standing Medical Advisory Committee. *Blood cholesterol testing: the cost-effectiveness of opportunistic cholesterol testing*. Report to the Secretary of State for Health, May 1990, London.

Wilkin, D. and Smith, A. (1987). Variation in general practitioners' referrals to consultants. *Journal of the Royal College of General Practitioners* **37**, 350–3.

Hall, D.M.B. (1989). *Health for all children — a programme for child health surveillance.* Oxford University Press, Oxford.

13 The effectiveness of referral guidelines: a review of the methods and findings of published evaluations

Ian Russell and Jeremy Grimshaw

Introduction

In Chapter 12 Haines and Armstrong describe how referral guidelines are being developed in British general practice. In this chapter we ask how effective such guidelines are in improving the referral of patients. After defining 'evaluation', we consider the criteria by which the effectiveness of guidelines might be judged. We describe the research designs available to evaluate whether guidelines are effective when judged by those criteria.

We then review the literature on the effectiveness of guidelines. Unfortunately we have identified only one published evaluation of guidelines specifically for referral — De Vos Meiring and Wells (1990). We therefore expand our review to include other evaluations of clinical guidelines. Foremost among these supplementary evaluations is the North of England Study of Standards and Performance in General Practice (1992); although this study was concerned with condition-specific guidelines for the care of children within general practice, the guidelines all give advice on referral.

All but one of the evaluations we review suggest that clinical guidelines are effective, but not in all circumstances. To discriminate between circumstances which are more or less favourable we suggest a taxonomy for such guidelines. By classifying the known evaluations within this taxonomy, we derive recommendations for the future use and evaluation of clinical guidelines.

What is evaluation?

In this chapter we use 'evaluation' to describe the process of choosing between alternative health care policies by identifying, measuring, and if possible by valuing the advantages and disadvantages of each (Russell 1983). This process can be broken down into three main stages. Firstly, we identify all the resources likely to be consumed, and the benefits likely to be generated, by each of the alternative policies. Table 13.1, derived from

Table 13.1 *North of England Study of Standards and Performance in General Practice: summary of incremental costs and benefits of comprehensive guidelines for selected conditions (Russell* et al. *1990a).*

To whom?	Costs	Benefits
General practitioner trainers	Time devoted to developing guidelines	Improvements in knowledge and job satisfaction
General practitioners	Time devoted to implementing guidelines	
Patients with selected conditions	Change in pattern and cost of care	Change in clinical and social outcomes of care
Other patients	Change in number and length of consultations	Indirect changes in appropriateness of diagnosis and management
Rest of the NHS	Change in cost of drugs, investigations and referral to hospital	Improvement in training of future general practitioners

Russell *et al.* (1990*a*), shows how this was done in the North of England Study. Note that 'benefit' is no more than a synonym for 'advantage' and that few of the costs listed are financial; they are better described as 'opportunity costs' in the sense that each represents the loss of an opportunity to use resources in some other way (Drummond 1980). Note too that Table 13.1 aims to estimate only the incremental benefits and costs of the change in policy to be evaluated, rather than the total benefits and costs of the health care activity in question.

The second stage in the process of evaluation is to estimate the magnitude of the incremental benefits and costs thus identified. The key issue here is to identify a research design which will enable us to draw robust scientific conclusions when we seek to attribute the changes observed to the policy being evaluated. There is a great danger that the observed changes have been caused not by the change of policy but by a simultaneous change in another influential variable. As an example, those who sought to attribute the fall in the prevalence of tuberculosis to the introduction of the BCG vaccine were thwarted by many synchronous changes, for example in the effectiveness of tuberculosis therapy (Cochrane 1989). Another major danger is that of confusing cause with effect. As an example, the Governor of Connecticut attributed the fall in road traffic deaths within that state in the early months of 1956 to the strict anti-speeding campaign which he had instigated at the beginning of that year; but the elegant mathematical analysis reported by Campbell and Ross (1968) could not rule out the alternative explanation that the anti-speeding campaign was no more than a response to a peak in road traffic deaths in the last quarter of 1955, a peak that would have subsided whether or not there had been any campaign.

Ideally, the final stage in the process of evaluation is to put values on as many as possible of the estimated benefits and costs of the policy under review, with a view to facilitating the decision whether to introduce this policy more widely. Suppose that evaluation were to show that referral guidelines for dyspepsia increase the numbers both of patients referred with moderate to severe abdominal problems who can benefit from secondary care and of patients with mild dyspepsia whose referral is generally considered inappropriate; how does one decide whether the guidelines have improved the quality of referral decisions? We know of only one study of referrals from general practice that has succeeded in putting values on all the estimated benefits and costs of a new policy; Russell *et al.* (1978) showed that a proposal to disperse outpatient clinics from a district general hospital in Carlisle to peripheral locations like Penrith would have generated benefits to patients worth little more than the cost to the NHS of dispersing these clinics. Despite the growing literature devoted to the economic appraisal of health care (Drummond *et al.* 1986), however, the valuation of benefits and costs is still very difficult, at least within the field of general practice. Fortunately a successful outcome to the second stage of evaluation, in the form of a complete table of the estimated benefits and costs, represents a powerful aid to decision-making and therefore a legitimate goal for evaluators.

Criteria for evaluation

Donabedian (1966) proposed three criteria by which the quality of medical care might be evaluated:

1. Structure — the resources available to the doctor whose care is being evaluated (including equipment and drugs, and also his own skills and training).

2. Process — what that doctor does to or for the patient.

3. Outcome — the resulting changes in the health of that patient.

Although Donabedian acknowledged the theoretical superiority of patient outcomes he argued that they were difficult to measure and limited in their application. In his view measures of process were more relevant to the question of whether medicine was properly practised. But he was rightly suspicious of the lack of evidence showing that improvements in structure lead to improvements in outcome or even process.

Donabedian's initial preference for process evaluation was soon challenged, notably by Deniston *et al.* (1968) and Greenberg (1968). Later a consensus emerged which has persisted ever since; whenever possible, outcome studies should measure process (Brook *et al.* 1977) and process studies should measure outcome (Donabedian 1980). Dissension in the 1960s gave way to consensus in the 1980s because both camps realized that their approach was flawed and needed to be strengthened. Process evaluators became increasingly aware that little of current medical practice had been established as effective by rigorous scientific methods (Cochrane 1989). To validate their process measures they began to include outcome measures in their evaluations. As an example, Hulka *et al.* (1979) incorporated measures of outcome for diabetes, hypertension, and urinary tract infection in the design of a typical process evaluation.

Outcome evaluators encountered practical problems of two basic types. Fistly, there were problems of attribution similar to those discussed on page 180. Suppose, for example, that the Grampian Referral Initiatives Project (Russell *et al.* 1990*b*; Ruta *et al.* 1990) were to generate robust scientific evidence that a combination of condition-specific referral guidelines developed by consultants, and discussions between consultants and GPs about referral for the same conditions, had improved health outcomes for patients; how could we disentangle beneficial effects arising from referral guidelines from those arising from discussions? Although our research design is sufficiently powerful to provide some information on this question, we have also kept records of all the meetings devoted to drawing up guidelines and tape-recordings of all the discussions between consultants and practitioners. Only in this way shall we be able to derive the most from our evaluation. Many other outcome evaluators have recognized that the collection of process data can greatly enhance their chances of drawing robust scientific conclusions.

Outcome evaluators were also persuaded to measure process by the very problems of measuring outcome. A major problems is that of *validity*; does the measure provide an accurate assessment of some aspect of patients' health or welfare? As an example, does blood sugar provide a valid measure of the effectiveness of referral for diabetes? Can it be regarded as an *intermediate outcome* in the sense that it predicts future complications like retinopathy and peripheral vascular disease? Another major problem is that of *reliability*; does the measure yield comparable assessments when used on different occasions by the same observer, or by different observers on the same occasion? As an example, do post-operative wound infections provide a reliable measure of the effectiveness of referral for benign lumps? Are they recorded consistently by different health professionals or even different individuals within the same profession? Practical tools for improving validity and reliability are summarized by Streiner and Norman (1989).

Validity and reliability are not the only problems to be overcome. As an example, recurrence rate is a valid and reliable measure of the effectiveness of referral for inguinal hernia. Yet if we measure recurrence 12 months after surgery there will be so few events that our measure will be lacking in *precision*. But if we measure recurrence 10 years after surgery (as many surgeons recommend) our measure will be lacking in *timeliness*. In this example there is a potential solution to the problems of precision and timeliness; recurrence could be measured by successive annual postal questionnaires to patients without much loss of validity or reliability.

For these reasons and more, those who seek to evaluate alternative health care policies should give equal weight to process and outcome criteria. Even structure criteria have an important role in pinpointing professionals or patients who are more or less likely to benefit from these policies. In short, health care evaluation should be based on a comprehensive package of criteria covering patient outcomes, health care activities, and health care resources. As an example Table 13.2 summarizes the data collected by the North of England Study (1990*b*) to evaluate comprehensive guidelines for recurrent wheezy chest in children. Although many components of this package suffer from problems of measurement, the complete package is greatly strengthened by the many interrelationships between these components. Thus it provides a robust and comprehensive set of criteria for evaluating changes in care, including referral guidelines.

Designs for evaluation

There are three basic research designs for evaluating alternative health care policies. Firstly, we can conduct a scientific experiment; we change the status quo specifically to compare alternative policies. Patients or doctors are allocated at random to new or existing policies. As an example, we could disseminate referral guidelines to a random sample of practices within a health district and compare the subsequent referral behaviour of that sample with that of the remaining practices.

Secondly, we can undertake a 'quasi-experimental' study; we behave *as if* we are conducting an experiment when in reality the status quo has been changed for some other reason. As an example, if a hospital disseminates referral guidelines to all practices within its catchment area then we could compare their subsequent referral behaviour with that of all practices within the catchment area of a hospital which has undertaken no dissemination. Although the typical quasi-experiment is opportunistic, evaluators can adopt this approach when there are practical or ethical barriers to conducting a genuine experiment. As an example, if the recommendations of a consensus conference are to be disseminated

Table 13.2 *North of England Study of Standards and Performance in General Practice: summary of data collected to evaluate comprehensive guidelines for recurrent wheezy chest in children (North of England Study 1990b).*

Criterion	Document	Typical data
Structure	Practice questionnaire	Environment, population, organization, staff, policies, equipment, and record system
	Doctor questionnaire	Age, qualifications, continuing education, and commitments outwith practice
Process for guidelines	Trainer interview schedule	Process and value of developing and implementing clinical guidelines
Process for recurrent wheezy chest	Enhanced medical record	1. Formulation of problem with justification 2. Management decisions with reasons (both abstracted according to manual specifying data elements relevant to primary care of child with recurrent wheezy chest)
Process in general	Practice activity record	Patient — age, housing, reason for consulting Process — procedures, referral, length of consultation (both recorded for all consultations during specified week)
	Surgery record	1. Length of all surgeries and clinics 2. Numbers of patients attending or visited at home (both recorded for all activities during specified week)
Outcome	Postal questionnaire to parents	Patient — medical history Outcomes — clinical: for example, breathlessness; functional: for example, sleeping; psychological: for example, anxiety; educational: for example, drug compliance
	Parent interview schedule	Expanded version of postal questionnaire with extra sections on family background, perceptions of consultation, and social and economic costs of recurrent wheezy chest

through the press, no experiment is possible. But we can still treat the conference as an innovation; referral behaviour after the conference can be compared with that before.

Thirdly, we can observe the status quo if the policies to be compared can be observed without intervention. This is rarely possible when evaluating referral guidelines. But the observational approach has been adopted (with varying degrees of success) in the evaluation of such policies as hospital confinement for normal deliveries (Ashford *et al.* 1973), water fluoridation (Oldham and Newell 1977), and augmented home care as an alternative to hospital care for elderly people (Gibbens *et al.* 1982).

Observational studies

The fundamental problem of observational studies is that the populations to be compared may differ in characteristics which affect the outcomes being measured — characteristics other than the policies to be compared. If these differences are not known to the evaluator, nothing can be done to ameliorate the resulting bias. Even when these differences are known it is rarely possible to correct the resulting bias with any confidence. Although there are epidemiological and statistical techniques for tackling this problem (Armitage and Berry 1987) they suffer from one major disadvantage; in correcting the bias arising from the differing characteristics of the two samples these techniques are likely to distort the true difference in outcome between the two policies.

As an example, the prevalence of cancer in the 10 largest American cities with fluoridated drinking water was once substantially greater than in the 10 largest American cities with unfluoridated drinking water. Oldham and Newell (1977), commissioned to evaluate whether this difference was attributable to fluoridation, soon discovered that the two populations differed substantially in age, gender, and race, and that the inhabitants of the fluoridated cities were thereby at greater risk of cancer. By standardization (Armitage and Berry 1987) they were able to show that the imbalance in cancer prevalence could be entirely explained by the known imbalance in cancer risk. This enabled them to describe the claim that fluoride causes cancer as 'not proven'. However, their observational data could not justify the stronger statement that fluoride does not cause cancer, because they could never be sure that the risk of cancer within their two populations did not differ in other, unknown ways.

Quasi-experimental studies

Although quasi-experiments take many forms (Cook and Campbell 1979), health care evaluators have rarely looked beyond the before-and-after design; the study population experiences one of two policies in the first phase, and the other in the second phase. Since many characteristics of the study population will be identical in both phases, this design is superior to that of observing the status quo. Nevertheless, the before-and-after design can still be fatally undermined by secular trends or sudden changes, either in the outcomes to be measured or in character-istics of the study population that influence those outcomes. Examples of these dangers are given on pages 180 and 181.

To ameliorate these problems it is prudent to identify a control popu-lation which will experience both the existing policy throughout the study period, and trends and changes similar to those of the study population. In evaluating the Connecticut anti-speeding campaign, for example, Campbell and Ross (1968) used data from the adjacent states of Massachusetts, New Jersey, New York, and Rhode Island. Even with such a control population, however, the evaluator faces the difficult task of monitoring all the differences between the study and control populations that could bias his evaluation — a task that few evaluators discharge convincingly (Russell 1983).

Experimental studies

Many eminent authorities, notably Cochrane (1989) and Hill and Hill (1991), have argued that the only safe method of avoiding the biases inherent in observational and quasi-experimental studies is by conducting a randomized trial. Their argument is almost as relevant to guidelines as to other health care innovations. However, there is one difference; it is difficult to allocate the successive patients of an individual doctor at random between guideline and control groups, since he or she may be influenced by the guidelines when deciding how to manage control patients. At first sight the solution to this problem is simple; doctors should be randomized rather than patients.

The change from randomizing patients to randomizing doctors has two important implications. Firstly, the calculation of the sample size needed to achieve an acceptable statistical power (for example, Russell 1984) becomes even more critical, since doctors are more difficult to recruit than patients. Secondly, there is a real danger of bias if the design is that of a simple randomized trial in which doctors are allocated at random between guideline and control groups. Our previous experience (North of England Study 1990c) suggests that randomization to the guideline group would motivate doctors more than randomization to the control group; this beneficial effect of taking part in research is known to social scientists as the Hawthorne effect (Moser and Kalton 1971).

The most attractive solution to this problem is to create guidelines for at least two conditions or topics. This enables each doctor to receive guidelines for one condition while acting as a control for another, thus enjoying the same Hawthorne effect as other participants. The statistical term for an experimental design which fulfils this requirement is a

Table 13.3 *Grampian Referral Initiatives Project: 'Latin square' experimental design (Russell* et al. *1990b).*

Intervention	Study condition			
	Low back-pain	Menorrhagia	Suspected peptic ulcer	Varicose veins
Guidelines and discussion with consultants	Group A	Group B	Group C	Group D
Discussion without guidelines	Group B	Group C	Group D	Group A
Guidelines without discussion	Group C	Group D	Group A	Group B
Neither guidelines nor discussion	Group D	Group A	Group B	Group C

Example: The entry in the top right-hand cell shows that Group D (a random sample of eligible practitioners, stratified by locality and referral rate) received guidelines for varicose veins and met consultants who had developed those guidelines. By moving down the diagonal towards the bottom left-hand cell, we see that Group D also met consultants who had developed guidelines for suspected peptic ulcer, and received guidelines for menorrhagia, but experienced no intervention for low back-pain.

'balanced incomplete block' (Cochran and Cox 1957); 'balanced' indicates that each doctor is effectively acting as his or her own control, and 'incomplete' that he or she is not expected to manage both guideline and control patients for the same condition.

Both the North of England Study (1992) and the Grampian Referral Initiatives Project (GRIP) have successfully implemented an elegant balanced incomplete block design known as a Latin square (Cochran and Cox 1957). The GRIP design (Table 13.3) gives each participating GP the opportunity to work on four study conditions and to experience each of four interventions — referral guidelines, discussion with consultants about referral, both of these, and neither of these. As foreseen on page 182, this design will also help to disentangle beneficial effects arising from referral guidelines from those arising from discussions. While we encourage potential evaluators to exploit this and other advantages of the Latin square, we recognize that many can only evaluate the introduction of referral guidelines as a complete package. Given how little is known about the effectiveness of referral guidelines, all such evaluations will be very welcome!

Finally, one caveat is needed about balanced incomplete block designs; the behaviour of participating practitioners may be contaminated, either by contact with other participants, or if a guideline for one condition influences the management of another condition. Fortunately, unlike the Hawthorne effect, such contamination is conservative; it underestimates the true effect of guidelines on the process and outcome of medical care.

Published evaluations of guidelines

We know of only one evaluation of guidelines specifically for referral — De Vos Meiring and Wells (1990). We therefore expand this review to cover evaluations of other types of guideline. In doing so we recognize one potential difference; referral guidelines should be as concerned to avoid under-referral as over-referral, while other guidelines are typically concerned to reduce overuse. But there are obvious exceptions to this generalization; De Vos Meiring and Wells (1990) were keen to reduce referrals to radiology, and the North of England Study (1990*a*) was keen only to improve the quality of child care in general practice. Furthermore, those who use and evaluate referral guidelines should beware of the temptation to adopt referral rates as their sole criterion of success; appropriateness of referral (Chapter 10) and patient outcome (pages 182–4) are equally relevant.

To keep our review relevant to the topic of referral guidelines, we follow the definition proposed by Field and Lohr (1990) — systematically developed statements to assist practitioner decisions about appropriate health care for specific clinical circumstances. This excludes sets of criteria for the appropriateness of individual items of care that have not been integrated into coherent guidelines (for example, Hulka *et al.* 1979; Park *et al.* 1986), educational programmes which do not generate guidelines (reviewed by Haynes *et al.* 1984; White *et al.* 1989 provides a more recent example), and feedback on clinical performance which is not related to specific guidelines (reviewed by Mugford *et al.* 1991). Tables 13.4 and 13.5 summarize 11 published experimental evaluations of guidelines thus defined; the division between balanced incomplete block designs (Table 13.4) and simpler randomized trials (Table 13.5) reflects our belief that the former are much less at risk to the Hawthorne effect described on page 186. Table 13.6 summarizes four controlled before-and-after evaluations of guidelines as defined above.

Table 13.7 concludes this review by selecting from the many uncontrolled before-and-after evaluations three which were careful or fortunate enough to draw conclusions which seem valid enough to merit discussion. However, we have excluded the oft-quoted study by Lomas *et al.* (1989); in our view, they failed to overcome the considerable methodological difficulty inherent in an uncontrolled study. In making this judgement we are adopting an implicit criterion for including studies within our review. Those who undertake formal reviews ('meta-analysis') of evaluations of well-defined innovations in health care adopt even stricter criteria, typically by reviewing only randomized trials (Chalmers 1989; Koes *et al.* 1991). They are usually able to summarize all the reviewed evidence by a single statistic, for example a combined relative risk of mortality (Yusuf *et al.* 1985). Although no such summary is possible in this review, the tables which follow seek, where possible, to compare the studies they summarize by expressing the effect of guidelines on compliance in absolute percentages. In effect, they assume that an improvement from 10–20 per cent is no more or less important than an improvement from 50–60 per cent; both represent an absolute change of 10 per cent.

Complex randomized trials (Table 13.4)

Cohen *et al.* (1985) evaluated the circulation of published guidelines advocating a series of preventive procedures. Each of 80 residents received guidelines relating to half the preventative procedures while acting as a control for the guidelines relating to the remaining procedures. The guidelines generated 'modest' improvements in residents' knowledge of the preventative procedures and in their compliance with those procedures.

In a sequel to Cohen *et al.* (1985), Tierney *et al.* (1986) evaluated retrospective feedback on compliance with Cohen's guidelines, and prospective reminders about patients to whom Cohen's guidelines were appropriate. Each of 140 residents received feedback on their compliance with half the preventive procedures while acting as a control for feedback on compliance with the remaining procedures; each received reminders about half the preventive procedures while acting as control for reminders about the remaining procedures. The reminders generated a greater improvement in residents' compliance with the preventive procedures than did the feedback.

In the smallest of the studies we reviewed, Norton and Dempsey (1985) evaluated the effect of developing guidelines within a single family medicine teaching unit. One group of three physicians developed guidelines for the care of cystitis, while another group of three developed guidelines for vaginitis; each group acted as a blind control for the other. Each group showed a significant improvement in the management of their allocated condition but no significant change in the management of their control condition.

In a more ambitious study Palmer *et al.* (1985) evaluated guidelines for eight specified medical tasks — four within internal medicine and four within paediatrics. These guidelines were developed by groups of participants and compliance with them was monitored within 'the audit cycle' (Hughes and Humphrey 1990; Irvine and Irvine 1991). Each of 16 group practices undertook audits for two of the four tasks appropriate to their discipline and acted as a control practice for the other two tasks.

Table 13.4 *Evaluation of guidelines by complex randomized trials ('balanced incomplete block designs')*

Year	Authors	Context	Subject	Design	Effect (absolute percentages unless otherwise stated)
1985	Cohen, S.J. et al.	US internal medicine residency programme	Preventive care	Latin square — 2 groups of 80 residents × 2 sets of 6 preventive care actions × guidelines versus no guidelines	(1) Knowledge of guidelines (structure) increased by 9% — from 53% to 62% (2) 'Modest' increase in compliance with guidelines (process)
1985	Norton and Dempsey	Canadian family medicine teaching unit	Cystitis and vaginitis	Latin square — 2 groups of 3 physicians × 2 conditions × guidelines versus no guidelines	Developing guidelines improved participants' compliance for both conditions: (1) Cystitis by 28% — from 38% to 66% (2) Vaginitis by 9% — from 22% to 31%
1985	Palmer et al.	16 US primary care practices	4 medical and 4 paediatric tasks	Balanced incomplete block design — each practice received guidelines and feedback for 2 tasks, and acted as control for the other 2 similar tasks	Compliance with guidelines showed: (1) 10% increase for gastroenteritis care (2) 7% increase for well child care (3) No significant increase for remaining 6 tasks

Year	Study	Setting	Topic	Design	Results
1986	Tierney *et al.*	US internal medicine clinic	Preventive care	Balanced incomplete block design based on 2 × 2 factorial design — 4 groups of 30 residents × 2 sets of 6 preventive care protocols × reminder versus no reminder × feedback versus no feedback	(1) Reminders increased compliance by 15% — from 15% to 30% (2) Feedback increased compliance by 7% — from 15% to 22%
1991	North of England Study of Standards and Performance in General Practice	62 training practices	Care of children in general practice (including referral)	Replicated Latin square — 10 groups of 9 trainers × 5 symptomatic conditions × 5 types of medical audit (including developing guidelines)	Developing (but not receiving) guidelines improved: (1) GPs' compliance with guidelines for all 5 conditions (a) Antibiotic prescribing by 10% (b) Therapeutic prescribing by 7% (c) Follow-up by 6% (2) Outcome for 1 condition (recurrent wheezy chest): (a) Drug compliance by 14% (b) Breathlessness from 4.2–1.7 days/month

Table 13.5 *Evaluation of guidelines by simple randomized trials*

Year	Authors	Context	Subject	Design	Effect (absolute percentages unless otherwise stated)
1978	Morgan et al.	US prepaid health plan	Antenatal care	About 1000 patients randomized between experimental group (automatic computer-generated reminder) versus control group	Compliance with guidelines increased: (1) In experimental patients by 15% — from 83% to 98% — within six months (2) In control patients by 11% — from 83% to 94% — within 12 months
1978	Sanazaro and Worth	50 US hospitals reviewed by Professional Standards Review Organizations	7 conditions — 4 medical, 2 surgical, and 1 paediatric	24 experimental hospitals (where guidelines were endorsed by medical staff and inserted in patients' medical records) versus 26 control hospitals	(1) Compliance with treatment guidelines increased by 2% (statistically significant) (2) No significant change in compliance with documentation guidelines or intermediate outcomes
1980	Hopkins et al.	US surgical emergency department	Hypotensive shock	Experimental group of residents on 1 surgical team (who were instructed in use of guidelines) versus control group of residents on 2 other surgical teams	(1) Compliance with guidelines (process) increased from 19/42 (45%) to 40/49 (82%) (2) Patients needing ventilation (outcome) reduced from 12/36 (33%) to 6/44 (14%)

Year	Author	Setting	Topic	Study design	Results
1980	Linn	US hospital emergency department	Management of burns	11 experimental hospitals (which conducted educational programme including guidelines) versus 9 control hospitals	(1) Non-compliance with guidelines (process) reduced from 4.3–2.8 items on average (2) Patient compliance with treatment (intermediate outcome) increased by 20%
1982	Cohen, D.I. et al.	US medical outpatient department	Preventive care	2 experimental medical teams (for whom guidelines were attached to patients' medical records) versus 1 control medical team	(1) Attitudinal scores (structure) increased by 15% — from 48% to 63% (2) Compliance with guidelines (process) increased by 32% — from 4% to 36%
1985	Putnam and Curry	16 Canadian family practices	5 conditions — A and B selected by experimental group; C, D, and E by external group (E secretly)	Experimental group of 8 family doctors (who devised guidelines for B and D) versus control group of 8 family doctors	(1) Participation in selecting conditions A and B did not increase compliance with guidelines (2) Devising guidelines A and C increased compliance with 'optimal criteria' by 32% (3) Receiving guidelines B and D increased compliance with 'essential criteria' by 22%

Table 13.6 *Evaluation of guidelines by controlled before-and-after studies*

Year	Authors	Context	Subject	Design	Effects (absolute percentages unless otherwise stated)
1980	Lohr and Brook	US Professional Standards Review Organisation (PSRO)	6 respiratory conditions	Time-series of prescribing of injections for 24 months after implementation of guidelines controlled by all other prescribing within PSRO	(1) Prescribing of injections reduced by 60%, while all other prescribing increased by 3% (2) Compliance with minimal criteria for antibiotic prescribing increased for all 6 conditions by between 6% and 39%
1983	Thompson *et al.*	US prepaid health plan (PHP)	'Routine' physical examinations	Before versus after guidelines: use of chest X-rays (CXR) and multi-channel blood tests (MCBT) controlled by external data, for example National Ambulatory Care Survey	(1) Examinations with non-indicated CXR reduced by 24% while national usage remained constant (2) Examinations with non-indicated MCBT reduced by 21%

Year	Author	Setting	Topic	Method	Results
1986	Fowkes *et al.*	5 major surgical hospitals	Pre-operative chest X-rays (CXR)	Time-series of CXR use before, and for 12 months after, implementation of guidelines in 4 hospitals controlled by 5th hospital	At best, CXR use/100 operations reduced by: (1) 16% by utilization review committee (2) 15% by review of CXR requests by radiologists (3) 12% by feedback to consultants on CXR use (4) 8% by new CXR request form (5) 3% in control hospital (not significant)
1990	De Vos Meiring and Wells	All general practices within 1 Health District	Referral for radiological examination	Before versus after guidelines: use of 9 examinations targetted by guidelines controlled by 5 examinations not so targetted	Use of targetted examinations reduced by 28% while use of examinations not targetted reduced by 2% (both relative to baseline)

Table 13.7 *Evaluation of guidelines by uncontrolled before-and-after studies*

Year	Authors	Context	Subject	Design	Effects (absolute percentages unless otherwise stated)
1982	Rodney et al.	US family medicine residency programme	Screening for colorectal cancer	Before versus after implementation of guidelines	Use of sigmoidoscopy increased by 21% — from 1/144 to 21/100
1984	Fowkes et al.	Hospital accident and emergency department	Skull X-ray (SXR) in patients with head injuries	Time series of SXR use over 3 periods of 4 months — before, during, and after implementation of guidelines	(1) Use of SXR reduced by 51% — from 65/1000 new attenders to 32/1000 (process) (2) No significant change in admission for head injuries (intermediate outcome)
1987	Kosecoff et al.	US National Institute of Health Consensus Development Programme	(1) Breast cancer (2) Caesarean section (3) Coronary artery bypass grafting (CABG)	Surveys limited to Washington State — of medical records in 10 hospitals — before and after each of 4 consensus conferences	No significant acceleration in rate of increase in compliance with 11 recommendations from 4 conferences

Participants showed a significant improvement in compliance with the guidelines for only two of the eight tasks — a finding that the authors attributed to conflict between the internal quality-oriented guidelines and external pressures to constrain costs.

The North of England Study (1992) was equally ambitious; ten groups of GP trainers developed guidelines for five conditions of childhood — acute cough, acute vomiting, bedwetting, itchy rash, and recurrent wheezy chest (Table 13.2). All ten groups achieved significant changes in prescribing and follow-up, all in the direction advocated by their guidelines. The two groups who developed guidelines for recurrent wheezy chest also achieved a significant improvement in drug compliance and a spectacular improvement in patient outcome, reducing morbidity in the form of breathlessness and wheeziness by more than a half. Given the robust experimental designs adopted by these first five evaluations, they provide reliable evidence that guidelines are effective in improving some aspects of medical care.

Simple randomized trials (Table 13.5)

We suggested on page 186 that randomizing successive patients of an individual doctor between guideline and control groups carried a danger that the guidelines might influence the management of control patients. Because Morgan *et al.* (1978) wanted to test this hypothesis they deliberately chose to randomize patients between a control group and an experimental group for whom any non-compliance by the doctor generated an automatic reminder from the computer-based medical record system. Their findings are important for both the users and evaluaters of guidelines; compliance in experimental patients rose from 83–98 per cent within 6 months, while compliance in control patients rose from 83–94 per cent in 12 months.

In contrast we are concerned that the remaining five evaluations in Table 13.5 are all unknowingly at risk to the Hawthorne effect despite their use of randomization. Sanazaro and Worth (1978) disseminated guidelines for the care of seven conditions, ranging from gastroenteritis in children to acute myocardial infarct in adults, within 24 large hospitals selected at random out of 50. They were hard pressed to demonstrate any effects of doing so: there was no significant change in either compliance with criteria relating to record-keeping or in intermediate patient outcomes (page 182); but an increase of only 2 per cent in compliance with criteria relating to treatment proved, somewhat fortuitously, to be statistically significant.

Linn (1980) also disseminated guidelines to a randomly selected subset of a group of large hospitals. He arranged seminars on the management of burns, during which guidelines were disseminated, in 11 out of 20 hospitals. He found that subsequent compliance with these guidelines was better in the experimental hospitals. Since all patients are motivated to recover from illness we believe that they are less at risk to the Hawthorne effect than doctors. Thus it is reassuring that the improved doctor compliance with guidelines was validated by improved patient compliance with treatment.

Hopkins *et al.* (1980) set out to evaluate an existing local algorithm for the management of hypotension in surgical emergency patients. This algorithm was disseminated to one surgical team but not to another two. Analysis showed significant improvements in compliance with guidelines among residents in the experimental group and in the reported need for ventilation (an intermediate outcome — page 182) among their patients. However, there is still room for suspicion that these may have Hawthorne effects.

The same criticism can be levelled at a very similar study by Cohen *et al.* (1982). They tried to evaluate the attachment to medical records of previously published guidelines recommending a series of age-specific preventive procedures. Two general medical teams were allocated to the intervention group and one (or two — the paper is ambiguous) to the control group. Again analysis showed significant improvements in compliance among residents in the intervention group. But in the absence of corroboration the paper gives little confidence that this improvement can be attributed to the introduction of the guidelines rather than to the Hawthorne effect.

Putnam and Curry (1985) evaluated the development, dissemination, and implementation of clinical guidelines within 16 Canadian family practices. Although they did not adopt a balanced incomplete block design, they took many other steps to strengthen their simple randomized trial in the face of potential Hawthorne effects. Although participation in selecting conditions for guidelines had no effect on compliance, both participation in developing those guidelines and receiving guidelines developed by others had a substantial effect.

Controlled before-and-after studies (Table 13.6)

We believe that before-and-after studies which are controlled consistently in both phases (page 186) may be less at risk to Hawthorne effects than randomized trials which fail to take account of this potential bias. In this spirit Lohr and Brook (1980) evaluated the effectiveness of guidelines restricting the use of antibiotic injections for respiratory infections. These guidelines were drawn up by the New Mexico Professional Standards Review Organization and finalized only after comments had been solicited from physicians across the state. They were then disseminated to all physicians in the state together with notification that Medicaid claims not meeting the guidelines would not be reimbursed. The prescription of anti-biotic injections fell substantially over the next two years while that of other prescriptions hardly changed. The size of this change, and the way in which the guidelines were implemented, suggest that the change may indeed be attributed to the guidelines.

Thompson *et al.* (1983) evaluated the effectiveness of guidelines advising against the use of chest X-rays and multichannel blood tests within routine physical examinations. These guidelines were drawn up by the 'medical staff committee on prevention' of a large prepaid health plan, and disseminated through an intensive educational programme. The proportions of relevant patients undergoing chest X-rays or blood tests fell over the four years of the study; in contrast, national usage of chest X-rays within routine physical examinations showed no change over this period. The size of this change, the use of appropriate control data, and the authors' careful checking of their conclusions all give confidence that the changes can be attributed to the guidelines.

Fowkes *et al.* (1986) evaluated the effectiveness of national guidelines advising restraint in the use of preoperative chest X-rays, drawn up by the Royal College of Radiologists. They disseminated these guidelines in four different ways in four different hospitals and also monitored the use of preoperative chest X-rays in a fifth, control hospital. The proportion of patients undergoing such X-rays fell significantly in all four experimental hospitals, but not in the control hospital. That these changes followed close on dissemination of the guidelines gives confidence that the changes can be attributed to the guidelines.

De Vos Meiring and Wells (1990) sent guidelines advising on referral for specific radiological examinations to all 150 GPs within the catchment area of their district general hospital. They observed a substantial change in the use of these targetted examinations and little change in the use of the untargetted examinations. The size of the change, and the careful conduct of the study, suggest that the change may indeed be attributed to the guidelines.

Uncontrolled before-and-after studies (Table 13.7)

Finally, from the many evaluations based on uncontrolled before-and-after studies, we have selected three whose findings seem to have some validity. Rodney *et al.* (1982) set out to evaluate the effectiveness of providing both a flexible (rather than rigid) sigmoidoscope and an extensive educational programme in increasing compliance with existing family practice guidelines advocating sigmoidoscopy to screen for colorectal cancer. However, their failure to identify a control population represented a major flaw in their research design. Nevertheless, an overwhelming increase in the proportion of eligible patients undergoing sigmoidoscopy — from one out of 144 to 21 out of 100 — does provide some evidence that the new steps taken to implement the guidelines may have caused the increase.

Another before-and-after study in danger of being undermined by the absence of a control population was that conducted by Fowkes *et al.* (1984) to evaluate the effectiveness of national guidelines advising restraint in the use of skull X-rays following head injury. These guidelines, drawn up by the Royal College of Radiologists, were introduced into a large X-ray department in three distinct stages. The ensuing fall of one half in the use of skull X-rays following head injury was closely linked in time to the staged introduction of the guidelines. Despite the flawed research design, this finding does suggest that the guidelines may have been responsible for the fall.

Kosecoff *et al.* (1987) describe the use of an uncontrolled before-and-after study to evaluate the effectiveness of guidelines generated by national consensus conferences. Because such guidelines are disseminated nationally there is little scope for identifying an appropriate control population. The only alternative is to conduct an uncontrolled study with the utmost scientific rigour. In evaluating the effectiveness of four separate American consensus conferences Kosecoff *et al.* (1987) conducted a rigorous survey of ten randomly selected hospitals in the State of Washington. Equally rigorous statistical analysis showed that compliance with the guidelines had increased since the conferences; however, the rate of increase was generally lower after the conferences than before, suggesting that the conferences had had no effect on medical practice. Nevertheless, the methods used by this evaluation can be questioned in one respect; given the inherent weakness of an uncontrolled before-and-after study, it is arguable that the study should have used more than one research method in more than one of the 50 American states.

Methodologically the 18 papers we have reviewed range from sound to suspect. All but Kosecoff *et al.* (1987) — the only one concerned with consensus conference guidelines — provide some evidence that guidelines are effective in improving medical care in some circumstances. To identify those circumstances more precisely we now suggest a tentative taxonomy for clinical guidelines.

A taxonomy for guidelines

The successful introduction of clinical guidelines is dependent on many factors including the clinical context and the methods of developing, disseminating, and implementing those guidelines. From our review we judge that different methods are appropriate in different contexts. Studies which report large improvements in clinical care suggest the true potential of guidelines when development, dissemination, and implementation are all appropriate. Studies which report small improvements or none may reflect failure at any stage during the introduction or evaluation of the

Table 13.8 *A taxonomy for clinical guidelines*

Probability of being effective (ceteris paribus)	Development strategy	Dissemination strategy	Implementation strategy
High	Internal	Specific educational intervention	Patient-specific reminder at time of consultation
Above average	Intermediate	Continuing medical education	Patient-specific feedback
Below average	External — local	Mailing targetted groups	General feedback
Low	External — national	Publication in professional journal	General reminder

guidelines. The main challenge for future evaluation is to specify which methods are appropriate in which circumstances.

Strategies for developing guidelines

Three issues seem to influence whether the development of guidelines is successful — how they are developed, by whom, and in what style. Tables 13.9 and 13.10 show that the methods used to develop guidelines include literature reviews (for example, Sanazaro and Worth 1978), small groups (for example, North of England Study 1990*a*), Delphi techniques (for example, Hulka *et al.* 1979), and consensus conferences (for example, Kosecoff *et al.* 1987). From the published evidence it is difficult to draw conclusions about which method is appropriate in which circumstances. In many studies the method of development is not described in detail. In others it is impossible to estimate the effectiveness of a method in the face of unsatisfactory dissemination, implementation, or evaluation.

As an example, in evaluating consensus conference guidelines Kosecoff *et al.* (1987) reported little change in medical practice. However, little effort had been devoted to dissemination or implementation. We conclude that guidelines developed by consensus conferences are not very effective in the absence of effective dissemination and implementation strategies. But we cannot estimate whether such guidelines would be effective with better dissemination and implementation.

Secondly, guidelines may be: *internal*, i.e. developed only by those who are to use them (for example, Norton and Dempsey 1985; North of England Study 1992); *intermediate*, i.e. developed by a group that includes representatives of those who are to use them (for example, Thompson *et al.* 1983; Palmer *et al.* 1985); or *external*, i.e. developed without those

Table 13.9 *Characteristics of guidelines evaluated in Tables 13.4 and 13.5*

Year	Authors	Type	Method of development	Method of dissemination	Method of implementation
1985	Cohen, S.J. et al.	External local	Abstracted from published guidelines	Internal mail	Credit at university bookshop after reading
1985	Norton and Dempsey	Internal	2 small groups	None	Feedback of data on baseline compliance
1985	Palmer et al.	Intermediate	2 small groups comprising 1 representative per practice plus researchers	Guidelines discussed, assessed, and then mailed	Feedback on compliance discussed and then mailed
1986	Tierney et al.	External local	Abstracted from published guidelines	Internal mail	(1) Computer-generated reminder in patients' medical records (2) Computer-generated monthly feedback on non-compliance
1992	North of England Study	Internal	10 small groups	Mailed to other groups	Feedback of data on baseline compliance

1978	Morgan et al.	External	American College of Obstetricians and Gynaecologists	Guidelines discussed at departmental meetings	Failure to comply caused computer-based medical record system to generate automatic reminder
1978	Sanazaro and Worth	External national	Literature review	Guidelines approved by medical staff	Copy of guidelines inserted at front of patients' medical records
1980	Hopkins et al.	External local	Small group	Residents instructed in use of guidelines for 30 minutes	Copy of guidelines carried by residents
1980	Linn	External national	Small group	Seminar lasting 4 hours focussing on guidelines	Copy of guidelines kept in emergency department
1982	Cohen, D.I. et al.	External local	Abstracted from published national guidelines	Series of five seminars on preventive medicine	Copy of guidelines attached to front of patients' medical records
1985	Putnam and Curry	2 internal and 3 external local	2 small groups — 1 internal (the experimental group) and 1 external	2 external guidelines mailed (3rd set of external guidelines kept secret)	(1) Interview to feed back data on baseline compliance (2) Subsequent personal educational package

Table 13.10 *Characteristics of guidelines evaluated in Tables 13.6 and 13.7*

Year	Authors	Type	Method of development	Method of dissemination	Method of implementation
1980	Lohr and Brook	Intermediate	Guidelines developed within PSRO and circulated outwith PSRO for comment	(1) Definitive guidelines mailed to all physicians (2) Physicians who had misused injectable drugs were visited	PSRO denied payment for Medicaid claims not complying with guidelines
1983	Thompson et al.	Intermediate	PHP medical staff committee on prevention	Extensive education programme over two years	Rates of CXR and MCBT within physical examination twice fed back to medical staff
1986	Fowkes et al.	External national	Royal College of Radiologists Working Party on Effective Use of Diagnositic Radiology	Guidelines approved by local divisions of radiology, anaesthetics, surgery, and gynaecology; and then sent to all consultants	(1) Utilization review committee, or (2) Review of CXR requests by radiology department, or (3) Feedback to consultants on use, or (4) New CXR request form

			Derived from guidelines developed elsewhere		
1990	De Vos Meiring and Wells	External local		Guidelines approved by Local Medical Committee and circulated by Family Practitioner Committee to all GPs	None — guidelines developed merely to advise GPs
1982	Rodney et al.	External national	American Cancer Society	Extensive educational programme	Introduction of flexible sigmoidoscope
1984	Fowkes et al.	External national	Royal College of Radiologists Working Party on Effective Use of Diagnostic Radiology	(1) Guidelines approved by senior staff (2) 2 seminars on guidelines	Introduction of structured head injury casualty card
1987	Kosecoff et al.	External national	4 national consensus conferences — 2 on breast cancer, and 1 each on caesarean section and CABG	(1) Publication in medical press (2) Mailed to relevant health professionals	None

who are to use them. External guidelines may be produced locally (for example, De Vos Meiring and Wells 1990; Russell *et al.* 1990*b*) or nationally (for example, Fowkes *et al.* 1986; Kosecoff *et al.* 1987).

Haines and Armstrong (Chapter 12) suggest that a sense of ownership is important if clinicians are to adopt guidelines. This is supported by the North of England Study (1992), which compared internal standards with external standards developed by local GPs; significant changes in process and outcome were apparent only for conditions for which participants had developed their own guidelines. However, studies evaluating intermediate or external guidelines have also observed significant changes in clinical behaviour (for example, Thompson *et al.* 1983; Fowkes *et al.* 1986). It seems that the greater the commitment of participants to the development of internal guidelines, the less the effort needed for dissemination and implementation.

Thirdly, there is little information in the literature about the effects of the format and style of guidelines on their adoption. On the basis of their previous experience, the North of England Study (Irvine *et al.* 1986) rejected 'deterministic' guidelines presented in the form of a fixed list of tasks in favour of 'branching' guidelines (for example, British Medical Journal 1989) in which the recommended course of action at each stage depends critically on the information available to the doctor. In their review of the guidelines produced by 24 national consensus conferences, Kahan *et al.* (1988) identified three different syles — scholarly (based on formal quantitative literature reviews), didactic (based on the work of expert groups), and consensual (based on the work of peer groups) — but they found no evidence on the relative effectiveness of these three styles.

Disseminating guidelines

Dissemination strategies are designed to ensure that target clinicians are aware of the guidelines. These strategies include publication in professional journals (for example, Kosecoff *et al.* 1987), mailing to targeted clinicians (De Vos Meiring and Wells 1990), continuing medical education (for example, Cohen *et al.* 1982), and specific educational initiatives. Our review suggests that the greater the educational component of the dissemination strategy, the greater the likelihood that the guidelines will be adopted into clinicians' practice. As an example, the success achieved by both Linn (1980) and Thompson *et al.* (1983) may be attributed with some confidence to their enthusiastic educational programmes, since neither devoted as many resources to development or implementation.

Strategies for implementing guidelines

Implementation strategies are designed to encourage clinicians to adopt the guidelines. These strategies fall into two groups, those which impinge on the structure of health care and those which are directed towards the process of care. Our review includes two examples of strategies affecting structure. Lohr and Brook (1980) observed a dramatic reduction in the prescription of injectable antibiotics when compliance with guidelines was linked to physician payment. Rodney *et al.* (1982) observed an equally dramatic increase in screening for colorectal cancer when new technology was introduced in the form of a flexible sigmoidoscope.

Implementation strategies directed towards process of care include general reminders (for example, guidelines kept available — Linn 1980), general feedback (for example, feedback on compliance with guidelines — Palmer *et al.* 1985), feedback specific to individual patients, and patient-specific reminders at the time of consultation. Our review includes two direct comparisons of different strategies. Fowkes *et al.* (1986) compared four different strategies for implementing guidelines for pre-operative chest X-rays — a utilization review committee, feedback to consultants, the introduction of a new X-ray form, and the screening of X-ray requests by radiologists; all these strategies were effective, but to varying degrees and for varying periods. Tierney *et al.* (1986) compared the effects of two strategies for improving compliance with preventive care protocols — monthly patient-specific feedback on non-compliance and patient-specific reminders at the time of consultation; they found that both strategies were effective but that reminders were better. Thus our review suggests that implementation strategies which are specific to individual patients are more likely to encourage clinicians to adopt guidelines.

Conclusions

The introduction of guidelines is a complex process with three crucial stages — development, dissemination, and implementation. Table 13.8 suggests a taxonomy for guidelines based on these three stages. Table 13.8 also summarizes our review of 18 published evaluations by identifying those strategies for development, dissemination, and implementation which seem to have a better chance of success; in simple terms, guidelines are more likely to be effective if they are developed by those who are to use them, if they are disseminated through education programmes designed for this purpose, or if they are implemented in conjunction with patient-specific reminders at the time of consultation.

Nevertheless, the evidence on the effectiveness of these strategies is sparse. The challenge to those who evaluate guidelines in future is to provide rigorous evidence on the relative effectiveness of different combinations of development, dissemination, and implementation strategies. It is also important to study the effect of factors like physical setting and clinical specialty. Our review has yielded encouraging evidence of the effectiveness of clinical guidelines. It suggests that an extended

programme of rigorous evaluation could bring substantial benefits to both
doctors and patients.

References

Armitage, P. and Berry, G. (1987). *Statistical methods in medical research* (2nd
edn). Blackwell, Oxford.

Ashford, J.R., Read, K.L.Q., and Riley, V.C. (1973). An analysis of variations
in perinatal mortality amongst local authorities in England and Wales.
International Journal of Epidemiology **2**, 31–46.

British Medical Journal (1989). Endocrine system: clinical algorithms. *British
Medical Journal*, London.

Brook, R.H., Avery, A.D., Greenfield, S. *et al.* (1977). Assessing the quality of
medical care using outcome measures: an overview of the method. *Medical Care*
15, Supplement.

Campbell, D.T. and Ross, H.L. (1968). The Connecticut crackdown on speeding:
time series data in quasi-experimental analysis. *Law and Society Review* **3**,
33–53.

Chalmers, I. (1989). Evaluating the effects of care during pregnancy and
childbirth. In *Effective care in pregnancy and childbirth: 1 — Pregnancy* (ed. I.
Chalmers M., Enkin, and M.J.N.C. Keirse). Oxford University Press, Oxford,
3–38.

Cochran, W.G. and Cox, G.M. (1957). *Experimental design* (2nd edn). Wiley, New
York.

Cochrane, A.L. (1989). *Effectiveness and efficiency: random reflections on health
services*. British Medical Journal for Nuffield Provincial Hospitals Trust, London.

Cohen, D.I., Littenberg, B., Wetzel, C., and Neuhauser, D.B. (1982). Improving
physician compliance with preventive medicine guidelines. *Medical Care* **20**,
1040–5.

Cohen, S.J., Weinberger, M., Hui, S.L., Tierney, W.M., and McDonald, C.J.
(1985). The impact of reading on physicians nonadherence to recommended
standards of medical care. *Social Science and Medicine* **21**, 909–14.

Cook, T.D. and Campbell, D.T. (1979). *Quasi-experimentation: design and analysis
issues for field settings*. Rand McNally, Chicago.

Denniston, O.L., Rosenstock, I.M., and Getting, V.A. (1968). Evaluation of
program effectiveness. *Public Health Reports* **83**, 323–35.

De Vos Meiring, P. and Wells, I.P. (1990). The effect of radiology guidelines for
general practitioners. *Radiology* **42**, 327–9.

Donabedian, A. (1966). Evaluating the quality of medical care. *Millbank
Memorial Fund Quarterly* **44**, 166–206.

Donabedian, A. (1980). *Explorations in quality assessment and monitoring: 1 —
The definition of quality and approaches to its assessment*. Health Administration Press, Ann Arbor, Michigan.

Drummond, M.F. (1980). *Studies in economic appraisal in health care*. Oxford
University Press, Oxford.

Drummond, M.F., Ludbrook, A., Lowson, K., and Steele, A. (1986). *Studies in
economic appraisal in health care — Volume 2*. Oxford University Press,
Oxford.

Field, M.J. and Lohr, K.N. (1990). *Clinical practice guidelines: direction of a new
agency*. Institute of Medicine, Washington DC.

Fowkes, F.G.R. *et al.* (1986). Multicentre trial of four strategies to reduce use of a radiological test. *Lancet* **i**, 367–70.

Fowkes, F.G.R., Williams, L.A., Cooke, B.R.B., Evans, R.C., Gehlbach, S.H., and Roberts, C.J. (1984). Implementation of guidelines for the use of skull radiographs in patients with head injuries. *Lancet* **ii**, 795–6.

Gibbens, F.J. *et al.* (1982). Augmented home nursing as an alternative to hospital care for chronic elderly invalids. *British Medical Journal* **284**, 330–3.

Greenberg, B.G. (1968). Evaluation of social programs. *Review of the International Statistical Institue* **36**, 260–77.

Haynes, R.B., Davis, D.A., McKibbon, A., and Tugwell, P. (1984). A critical appraisal of the efficacy of continuing medical education. *Journal of the American Medical Association* **251**, 61–4.

Hill, A.B. and Hill, I.D. (1991). *Bradford Hill's Principles of Medical Statistics* (Twelfth edn). Arnold, London.

Hopkins, J.A., Shoemaker, W.C., Greenfield, S., Chang, P.C., McAuliffe, T., and Sproat, R.W. (1980). Treatment of surgical emergencies with and without an algorithm. *Archives of Surgery* **115**, 745–50.

Hughes, J. and Humphrey, C. (1990). *Medical audit in general practice — a practical review of the literature*. Kings Fund Centre, London.

Hulka, B.S. *et al.* (1979). Peer review in ambulatory care: use of explicit criteria and implicit judgements. *Medical Care* **17**, Supplement.

Irvine, D.H. and Irvine, S. (1991). *Making sense of audit*. Radcliffe Medical, Oxford.

Irvine, D.H. *et al.* (1986). Performance review in general practice: educational development and evaluative research in the Northern Region. In *In pursuit of quality?* (eds D.A. Pendleton, T.P.C. Schofield, and M.L. Marinker) Royal College of General Practitioners, London.

Kahan, J.P., Kanouse, D.E., and Winkler, J.D. (1988). Stylistic variations in National Institutes of Health consensus statements, 1979–1983. *International Journal of Technology Assessment in Health Care* **4**, 289–304.

Koes, B.W., Assendelft, W.J.J., van der Heijden, G.J.M.G., Bouter, L.M., and Knipschild, P.G. (1991). Spinal manipulation and mobilisation for back and neck pain: a blinded review. *British Medical Journal* **303**, 1298–1303.

Kosecoff, J., Kanouse, D.E., Rogers, W.H., McCloskey, L., Winslow, C.M., and Brook, R.H. (1987). Effects of the National Institutes of Health consensus development program on physician practice. *Journal of the American Medical Association* **258**, 2708–13.

Linn, B.S. (1980). Continuing medical education: impact on emergency room burn care. *Journal of the American Medical Association* **244**, 565–70.

Lohr, K.N. and Brook, R.H. (1980). Quality of care in episodes of respiratory illness among Medicaid patients in New Mexico. *Annals of Internal Medicine* **92**, 99–106.

Lomas, J., Anderson, G.M., Dominick-Pierre, K., Vayda, E., Enkin, M.W., and Hannah, W.J. (1989). Do practice guidelines guide practice? The effect of a consensus statement on the practice of physicians. *New England Journal of Medicine* **321**, 1306–11.

Morgan, M., Studney, D.R., Barnett, G.O., and Winickoff, R.N. (1978). Computerised concurrent review of prenatal care. *Quality Review Bulletin* **4**, 33–6.

Moser, C.A. and Kalton, G. (1971). *Survey methods in social investigation* (Second edn). Gower, Aldershot.

Mugford, M., Banfield, P., and O'Hanlon, M. (1991). Effects of feedback of information on clinical practice: a review. *British Medical Journal* **303**, 398–402.

North of England Study of Standards and Performance in General Practice (1990*a*). *Final report: I — setting clinical standards within small groups.* Report 40. Health Care Research Unit, University of Newcastle upon Tyne.

North of England Study of Standards and Performance in General Practice (1990*b*). *Final report: II — methods for evaluating the setting and implementation of clinical standards.* Report 41. Health Care Research Unit, University of Newcastle upon Tyne.

North of England Study of Standards and Performance in General Practice (1990*c*). *Final report: III — the effects of setting and implementing clinical standards.* Report 42. Health Care Research Unit, University of Newcastle upon Tyne.

North of England Study of Standards and Performance in General Practice (1992). Medical audit in general practice. *British Medical Journal*, **304**, 1480–8.

Norton, P.G. and Dempsey, L.J. (1985). Self-audit: its effect on quality of care. *Journal of Family Practice* **21**, 289–91.

Oldman, P.D. and Newell, D.J. (1977). Fluoridation of water supplies and cancer — a possible association? *Applied Statistics* **26**, 125–35.

Palmer, R.H. *et al.* (1985). A randomised controlled trial of quality assurance in sixteen ambulatory care practices. *Medical Care* **23**, 751–70.

Park, R.E. *et al.* (1986). Physician ratings of appropriate indications for six medical and surgical procedures. *American Journal of Public Health* **76**, 766–72.

Putnam, R.W. and Curry, L. (1985). Impact of patient care appraisal on physician behaviour in the office setting. *Canadian Medical Association Journal* **132**, 1025–9.

Rodney, W.M., Quan, M.A., Johnson, R.A., and Beaber, R.J. (1982). Impact of flexible sigmoidoscopy on physician compliance with colorectal cancer screening protocol. *Journal of Family Practice* **15**, 885–9.

Russell, I.T. (1983). The evaluation of a computerised tomography: a review of research methods. In *Economic and medical evaluation of health care technologies* (eds A.J. Culyer and B. Horisberger). Springer-Verlag, Berlin.

Russell, I.T. (1984). Clinical trials and evaluation of surgical procedures. *Surgery* 196–9.

Russell, I.T. *et al.* (1990*a*). Performance review in British primary health care: an epidemiological and economic evaluation. In *Primary health care* (ed. P. Bergerhoff, D. Lehmann, and P. Novak). Springer-Verlag, Berlin.

Russell, I.T., Reid, N.G., Glass, N.J., and Akehurst, R.L., (1978). Cost benefit analysis in health services research: a case-study of the location of ambulatory care. *Proceedings of the Social Statistics Section of the American Statistical Association*, 167–172.

Russell, I.T., Taylor, R.J., and Grimshaw, J.M. (1990*b*). *Grampian Referrals Initiative Project: research proposal.* Health Services Research Unit, University of Aberdeen (mimeo).

Ruta, D.A. *et al.* (1990). *Grampian Health Outcomes Study: research proposal.* Health Services Research Unit, University of Aberdeen (mimeo).

Sanazaro, P.J. and Worth, R.M. (1978). Concurrent quality assurance in hospital care. *New England Journal of Medicine* **296**, 1171–7.

Streiner, D.L. and Norman, G.R. (1989). *Health measurement scales: a practical guide to their development and use.* Oxford University Press, Oxford.

Thompson, R.S., Kirz, H.L., and Gold, R.A. (1983). Changes in physician behaviour and cost savings associated with organisational recommendations on the use of routine chest X-rays and multichannel blood tests. *Preventive Medicine* **12**, 385–96.

Tierney, W.M., Hui, S.L., and McDonald, C.J. (1986). Delayed feedback of physician performance versus immediate reminders to perform preventive care. *Medical Care* **24**, 659–66.

White, P.T., Pharoah, C.A., Anderson, H.R., and Freeling, P. (1989). Randomised controlled trial of small group education on the outcome of chronic asthma in general practice. *Journal of the Royal College of General Practitioners* **39**, 182–6.

Yusuf, S., Peto, R., Lewis, J., Collins, R., and Sleight, P. (1985). Beta blockade during and after myocardial infarction: an overview of the randomized trials. *Progress in Cardiovascular Diseases* **27**, 335–71.

14 Hospital referral — the future

Martin Roland

For those who have grown up within the NHS it is easy to forget that the referral system has only existed in its present form since 1948. As Nigel Oswald describes in Chapter 2, the distinction between primary and secondary care was more blurred prior to 1948, and the constraints which operated on doctors earlier this century were very different to those which operate now. In particular, the establishment of a salaried service for hospital doctors and a secure financial base for quasi-independent GPs enabled boundaries to the delivery of care to be set which rapidly came to be accepted by doctors and which posed no threat to their financial security. Subsequently, the development of general practice into an identifiable discipline, particularly as a result of the changes following the 1964 GPs' Charter, enabled a relatively comfortable relationship to develop between GPs and consultants. GPs felt few constraints on whom they should refer to hospital, and specialists were protected from overwork by waiting-lists, which were the effective form of 'rationing' used in what has always been a cash-limited service.

However, the relatively recent development of the referral system as we know it emphasizes how sensitive the system is to structural change. It is therefore not surprising that the major changes in the NHS in 1991 have focused attention on hospital referrals. The fundamental change in the new NHS is the split between purchasers and providers, so each referral now becomes a financial cost either to the patient's HA or to their GP in the case of fundholders. The hospital service has always been the most expensive part of the NHS and therefore the hospital referral — as the principal means of accessing hospital care — is a natural focus of those seeking to ensure the most effective use of NHS resources.

The issue which has attracted the attention of health care planners is the variability that exists between GPs in their referral patterns. General practice is not unique in this respect. Variability in the delivery of medical care to apparently similar populations is one that perplexes planners across the world (well reviewed in a book by Andersen and Mooney 1990). In relation to hospital referral, government's attention was caught by a number of studies which apparently showed variation of up to 25-fold in the rates at which GPs refer patients to hospital. Although it now looks as if some of these very high figures may have been a result of the study of very small samples of referrals, there nevertheless probably exists at least a fourfold variation in true referral rates between GPs. The true extent and nature of this variability is likely to become clearer over the next few years with improving information about GPs' referral patterns. This will come partly from statutorily required data in GPs' annual reports, and partly from the development of improved information systems in NHS hospitals.

The reasons for the variability in referral patterns remain obscure. Research studies to date do not provide the explanation, though it may be that more detailed studies of the way in which doctors make clinical decisions will provide further clues. There has been very little work to back up theoretical models which have been advanced about how doctors make referral decisions. Furthermore, there has until very recently been an almost complete lack of studies looking at the outcome of different patterns of GP care. We do not know, for example, whether the GPs with high referral rates are profligate users of expensive hospital resources, thereby exposing their patients to inconvenience and potential risk. Alternatively, we do not know if the patients of the low-referring GPs are deprived of hospital resources from which they could benefit, and suffering as a consequence. Furthermore, we have no evidence to suggest that the 'average' referral rate is in any sense 'correct', or that the referrals of GPs with average rates of referral are any more appropriate than the referrals of their colleagues at the extremes of the distribution of referral rates.

In order for discussion about referral rates to progress meaningfully, it will be essential in future to look in much greater detail at the quality or appropriateness of referrals, and at the outcome of different types of referral. Furthermore, in looking at outcome it is important to realize that there are a range of relevant outcomes to referral decisions which include both clinical outcome and patient satisfaction. The need to meet patients' expectations is likely to become an increasingly important factor in referral decisions, particularly if patients' expectations of their health care system continue to grow.

When discussing 'quality' or 'appropriateness' in relation to hospital referral, it is important to realize that the various players in the field have different agendae illustrated in the following examples:

An unnecessary referral? (1)
The GP may regard as appropriate referral of a patient with a headache in whom he is concerned about the possibility of a brain tumour. The patient may regard the referral as unnecessary if he has no anxiety about his symptom, and the neurologist may regard the referral as inappropriate if his assessment of the probability of a brain tumour is very low.

An unnecessary referral? (2)
The GP may regard as of doubtful value the referral of a patient with occasional knee pain during competitive sport, where a change of sport would avoid the

problem and where a specialist is very unlikely to suggest any more than the physiotherapist has already done. The patient, however, enjoys his sport and wishes to leave no stone unturned before giving it up. The orthopaedic surgeon knows that he has no treatment to offer the patient and regards the patient as keeping him away from work where he could be of greater use to other patients.

An unnecessary referral? (3)

A middle-aged man with epigastric pain and weight loss is referred by his GP who fears a malignancy. He does not share this anxiety with the patient who is unconcerned about his symptoms. The specialist arranges an urgent gastroscopy which turns out to be normal, and the patient recovers. The patient considers that he has been exposed to unnecessary inconvenience and discomfort.

Many doctors feel uneasy with the language which starts to describe referrals as inappropriate, and are concerned about the implied threat to clinical freedom contained within discussions of which patients should, and which patients should not, be referred to hospital. However, such discussion makes explicit the rationing which has always existed in the NHS. Prior to 1990, the principal method of rationing was by the hospital waiting-list. The effect of high-referring doctors on the system was to increase the waiting-list for their own and for other doctors' patients. The 'rationing' becomes much more explicit for the patients of the GP fundholder, who has a direct choice on how to spread his budget over his population of patients. The budgets have been relatively unconstrained in the first year, allowing fundholders to purchase improved quality of care for their patients; for example, by buying care from the private sector and thereby short-circuiting waiting-lists. However, by establishing fundholding the government has developed a mechanism by which referrals may be cash-limited in future, and GPs may in a few year's time be faced with real and uncomfortable choices about which patients they can afford to refer. The government's view has been that rationing at primary care level is more appropriate than rationing by waiting-list as the GP is in the best position to prioritize the needs of his population.

Discussion of appropriateness of referral is therefore inevitable as our government, in common with those of all developed countries, puts increasing emphasis on value for money in health care. It is furthermore a discussion which British GPs will avoid to their cost. The evidence to date, sparse though it is, suggests that the great majority of referrals to hospital are appropriate. If one is seeking to explain the variation which exists in GP referral rates, it may be that the real 'problem' lies with GPs with low rates of referral to hospital. The referral system in this country limits the access of patients to specialists, and the British population receives less medical care from specialists (whether based in the community or in hospitals) than the populations of most Western European countries, and much less than those of the USA. If the issue of appropriateness of referral is addressed in detail, it may well be that substantial under-usage of specialist resources will be demonstrated. However, this will depend on developing methods of assessing referral based on the outcome of patients' care, and of addressing the outcome of patients not referred to hospital as well as those who are referred.

One aspect of the referral process that has been of recent interest is the development of referral guidelines. A number of groups around the country have developed guidelines to try and identify which patients would benefit most from hospital referral. The question of whether guidelines (in any circumstances) improve medical care is an open one. In Chapter 13 Russell and Grimshaw reviewed the evidence that practice guidelines affect clinical practice, and it is clear that their effectiveness is limited unless appreciable resources are put into the development, dissemination, or implementation of guidelines, in which case their cost-effectiveness may be questioned.

Doctors often find the concept of clinical guidelines threatening. They appear to strike at the heart of clinical freedom. The importance of clinical freedom depends to some extent on how it is used. If clinical freedom means the freedom to deliver inferior care, then clinical freedom is not something to which doctors should have an absolute right. How do guidelines fit into this debate, and how can guidelines contribute to patient care without threatening professional autonomy? Eddy (1990) makes a useful distinction between standards, guidelines, and options. Standards are so widely accepted that deviation from a standard would be very rare and difficult to justify (example of a standard: oral tetracycline should not be used in children). For a guideline, exceptions to the suggested management will be common and relatively easy to justify. A guideline should be developed on the basis of the known outcome of different treatments, and where the outcome of two management approaches may be similar, a guideline will suggest a choice in management (example: a number of interventions based in general practice have been shown to be effective in helping patients to stop smoking; for example, advice from the doctor or nurse, leaflets, and so on. Advice about smoking should therefore be available in practices). For options, there is little evidence on which to base any firm course of action, and a list of management alternatives may be all that can be provided. Development of guidelines and options is a powerful method of identifying areas of uncertainty which need to be acknowledged as such in order to prevent arbitrary management rules being proposed. These areas of uncertainty may then form the basis for future research.

One important effect of guideline development should be to draw GPs together with local specialists to discuss the local delivery of services, and improved dialogue between primary and secondary care doctors is likely to be valuable. These discussions need to take place at a local level. It is fairly clear that nationally-developed guidelines have relatively little effect if simply published in scientific journals; doctors (and not just GPs) do not change their clinical practice readily, and are rarely enthusiastic about doing so as a result of a guideline received through the post from a remote source with which they feel they have no involvement. However, local discussions between GPs and consultants offer the opportunity to try to match the clinical policies of local doctors with the needs of local populations and the local availability of resources.

One of the effects of the GP fundholding scheme is to stimulate dialogue between GPs and specialists, and indeed to explore new ways in which care may be delivered. Fundholders, ahead of other doctors, are exploring different ways of using specialists, and those which involve specialists working in GP surgeries are particularly likely to produce improved understanding about which patients will benefit most from specialist care. If these models are successful in fundholding practices, non-fundholders may wish to press DHAs to explore similar options on their behalf.

There are other ways in which our present model of the referral process might change in the future. One area where referrals appear to cause particular problems is in musculoskeletal medicine (orthopaedics and rheumatology), judged at least by the disproportionate number of papers published on referrals to these specialties. GPs are dissatisfied because their patients often wait for many months to see a specialist who sometimes can do little to improve the patient's disability. Orthopaedic surgeons are dissatisfied because they see many patients whose condition is not amenable to operative treatment. Some rheumatologists are happy to see soft-tissue injuries while others think that their skills are needed for patients with inflammatory joint disease. Interventions to improve GPs' skills in musculoskeletal medicine have been of limited effect, and patients are increasingly reluctant to accept limitation to the active lifestyle which their doctors have previously encouraged. It may be that an alternative model to the two-tier generalist/specialist model is needed for orthopaedics. A third tier of specialists in musculoskeletal medicine, who might be clinical assistants, could be interposed between the GP and the orthopaedic surgeon. If this sub-specialist saw patients in practices, he/she could increase GPs' confidence and skill with musculoskeletal problems, while at the same time referring on to orthopaedic surgeons only those patients who require surgery. Orthopaedic specialists do not appear to enjoy giving advice on non-operative treatment; they may not be very good at it. Perhaps it is time to relieve them of the burden.

This is an example of one of the ways in which the referral system could change in the future. In a time of rapid change in the NHS it seems unlikely that the system of hospital referrals which exists at present will remain unchanged. It is vital, however, that the changes which take place should do so on the basis of demonstrable improvement in patient outcome or demonstrable improvement in the efficiency with which hospital resources are used. Many of the questions about making the most effective use of hospital resources remain unanswered, and it is therefore appropriate that this book should end by looking forward to areas where research into hospital referral is needed in future.

An agenda for future research

There are many opportunities for further research into hospital referrals and this final section of the book identifies particular areas where further research is needed.

The decision to refer

Little work has been done to extend the two theoretical models which have been advanced to explain doctors' decisions about when to refer patients to hospital (Dowie 1983; Wilkin and Smith 1987). In particular, we need to know which elements of these models are related to the variation in response to possible referral scenarios that exists between GPs, or whether other elements not included in these models are important. It is likely that detailed descriptive analysis of doctors' decisions to refer, or not to refer, will be helpful in clarifying these models and identifying new elements to them. In particular, the way in which doctors respond to the context in which the referral decision is made may be important; for example, decisions made at the end of long surgeries, or when under particular time pressure. Another area which has received very little attention is the relationship between doctors' referral decisions and their actual clinical knowledge or skills. Work in this area, though clearly potentially threatening to doctors, could have important educational implications.

Decisions about and reasons for not referring patients to hospital are likely to be just as important as decisions to refer, and future work needs to include patients not referred to hospital as well as those referred. It may be that studying patients whom GPs identified as 'nearly referred' to hospital would be one feasible way to approach this issue.

One particular area which should be studied is the effect of fundholding on referral decisions. The ways in which fundholders make referral decisions are likely to be different from non-fundholders, not least because they may have available a different range of referral options. However, it will also be important to determine the extent to which fundholders are exposed to pressure not to refer patients who might benefit from referral.

Communication about referral

Communication — from GP to specialist and from specialist to GP — is a regular source of complaint. Both complain about the inadequacy of communication, but there seems to be considerable ambivalence about attempts to standardize information transfer so that, for example, the specialist would always be told about drugs the patient is on and about major illness in the patients' history, and that the GP would always be told about the specialist's management plan and what the patient has been told. A recent attempt to impose a nationally standardized format on a referral letter met, appropriately, with overwhelming resistance. Structures outlined for letters by carefully tailored software packages may have some role to play in the future, but the greatest impact of information technology is likely to be in speeding up the transfer of information, especially after discharge from hospital.

Minimum criteria for standards of communication may well be built into contracts in future, and indeed do form part of some fundholders contracts with provider units. One factor which may influence change in this area is the perceived need by specialists to have sufficient information on which to prioritize requests for referral; it may become more difficult for GPs to obtain early appointments unless an agreed set of data is provided. Future work in this area is likely to include developmental work to show possible models of good practice.

Referral rates

Variation in referral rates will continue to be an area of concern to managers. A system of feedback of referral rates has become institutionalized through GP Annual Reports, and there is concern that this will lead to a downward pressure on referral without any clear idea about the consequences on patient care. There is indirect evidence to suggest that quality of care is unrelated to referral rates, but this work needs to be extended in order to determine whether referral rates are a suitable target for managerial concern, or whether, as seems more likely, the focus needs to be on appropriate standards of care and on patient outcome. In the absence of such work, referral rates will continue to occupy a position of importance which is probably inappropriate and which results principally from the ease with which they may be measured.

Benefit from referral

The issue of appropriateness or quality of referrals can be guaranteed to raise professional hackles, particularly if clinical freedom appears to be threatened. Nevertheless, if some patients derive greater benefit from referral than others then it is a legitimate aim of providers to maximize the benefit which can be derived from limited resources.

Studies of the appropriateness of referral need to recognize the differing needs and perspectives of the GP, the specialist, and the patient, and need also to recognize that there is a distinction between medical appropriateness (for example, which patients with rectal bleeding should be referred to hospital) and societal decisions about what our health service can afford (for example, should sterilizations be reversed and can we afford arthroscopy of the knee in people experiencing minor limitation of amateur sporting activity?).

Central to assessment of the benefit of referral is the development of methods of measuring the outcome of referrals. The development of methods of outcome measurement suitable for use in primary care (Wilkin *et al.* 1992) should facilitate studies which seek to look at health gain in relation to hospitalization. However, studies of the benefits of referral need to be balanced by studies of patients with similar conditions who are not referred to hospital and who might have benefited from referral. It is much easier to look at patients referred to hospital than to look at their unreferred counterparts. The two groups are of essence unlikely to be comparable, and the ideal way to determine the benefit of referral would be to conduct randomized controlled trials of referral. Such trials, though theoretically desirable, are practically and ethically unfeasible. Under-referral might, however, be approached by randomized controlled trials offering specialist opinion about patients who had not been referred to hospital. Apart from randomized trials, comparisons of referred and unreferred patients will need to depend on longitudinal follow up of both types of patient, taking as much care as possible to identify and to quantify differences between the groups at the start. The most promising conditions on which to try this type of approach would be those where the benefit of hospital referral is doubtful — for example, back pain — or one where alternative practice based models of care might be offered — for example, benzodiazepine dependence.

Costs of referral

The financial consequences of variation in referral patterns will continue to be an important political issue for the foreseeable future. The financial costs of referral are only one of the 'costs' that need to be assessed in relation to referral. Other costs include the risk of unnecessary procedures being carried out and the opportunity cost of an 'inappropriate' referral to someone else who could have taken that patient's place in the clinic.

However, analysis of the costs of referrals has been relatively unsophisticated, and in particular has tended to carry the assumption that all referrals cost the same. This may not be the case. As an example, a referral which is regarded as inappropriate by an orthopaedic surgeon may generate no investigation or treatment costs, and may therefore be much less expensive than a referral of a patient requiring operation. More sophisticated hospital information systems may allow the relationship between referral rates and actual costs of referral to be explored in the fairly near future. It is certainly not automatic that a reduction in the number of referrals would reduce costs. If one imagines a scenario where all patients referred to orthopaedic clinics were put on operative waiting-lists, the outpatient waiting-list might decrease, but the inpatient waiting-list would increase. Rationing by waiting-list would still exist, but at a different stage in the system, and the reasons for the rationing would become more explicit. Future research into the costs of referrals should take issues such as these into account.

Referral guidelines

There is considerable enthusiasm at present for the development of referral guidelines in the expectation that they might either increase appropriateness of referral or reduce referral costs. Several authors in this book have pointed out that these expectations are at best hopeful and at worst improbable. Nevertheless, there is value in developing referral guidelines particularly for the contact between specialists and GPs in the development of guidelines. The taxonomy of guidelines proposed by Russell and Grimshaw in Chapter 13 suggests that there are three distinct issues to be addressed; how guidelines are developed, how they are disseminated, and what is done to facilitate their implementation. These three subjects are all fertile areas for research, and the evaluation of guidelines is likely to be an important area for research into hospital referrals in the next decade.

Conclusion

There have been substantial changes in the way in which care has been delivered over the last 20 years, including a major shift towards the management of chronic diseases like hypertension and diabetes in general practice, an increased emphasis on preventive care, appointment of nurse specialists both in primary and secondary care, to the most recent moves towards minor surgery being carried out in general practice. These and future changes are likely to continue to alter the relationship between GPs and hospital doctors, and it is important that the effects of such changes on the process, outcome, and costs of providing care should be measured.

The next few years are likely to be a time when those who have ideas about developing the interface between primary and secondary care will be able to find support and financial backing for experimental development projects. The bureaucratic notion that GP referrals to hospital are a 'problem' should be seen as a challenge to demonstrate where GPs are already providing excellent care, and where that care could be improved in future.

References

Andersen, T.F. and Mooney, G. (1990). *The challenges of medical practice variations*. Macmillan Press, London.

Dowie, R. (1983). *General practitioners and consultants: a study of outpatient referrals*. King's Fund, London.

Eddy, D.M. (1990). Designing a practice policy: standards, guidelines and options. *Journal of the American Medical Association* **263**, 3077–84.

Wilkin, D. and Smith, A.G. (1987). Explaining variation in general practitioner referrals to hospital. *Family Practice* **4**, 160–9.

Wilkin, D., Hallam, L., and Doggett, M-A. (1992). *Measures of need and outcome for primary health care.* Oxford University Press, Oxford.

Index